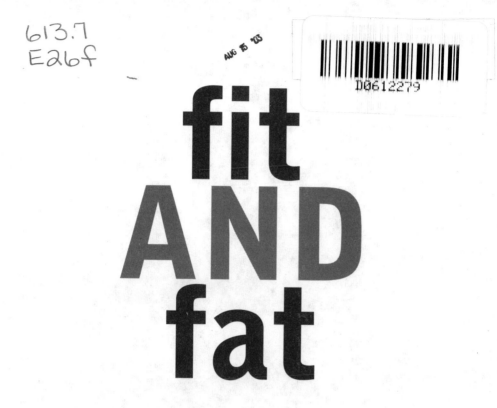

fit
AND
fat

fit AND fat

The 8-Week Heart Zones Program

SALLY EDWARDS

spokesperson for the Danskin® Women's Triathlon

AND LORRAINE BROWN

ALPHA

A member of Penguin Group (USA) Inc.

International Standard Book Number: 0-02-864423-9
Library of Congress Catalog Card Number: 2003100702

05   04   03   8   7   6   5   4   3   2   1

Interpretation of the printing code: The rightmost number of the first series of numbers is the year of the book's printing; the rightmost number of the second series of numbers is the number of the book's printing. For example, a printing code of 03-1 shows that the first printing occurred in 2003.

Printed in the United States of America

Publisher's note: Every effort as been made to ensure that the information contained in this book is complete and accurate. However, neither the publisher nor the authors is engaged in rendering professional advice or services to the individual reader. The ideas, procedures, and suggestions contained in this book are not intended as a substitute for consulting with your physician. All matters regarding your health require medical supervision. Neither the authors nor the publisher shall be liable or responsible for any loss or damage allegedly arising from any information or suggestion in this book.

Trademarks: All terms mentioned in this book that are known to be or are suspected of being trademarks or service marks have been appropriately capitalized. Alpha Books and Penguin Group (USA) Inc. cannot attest to the accuracy of this information. Use of a term in this book should not be regarded as affecting the validity of any trademark or service mark.

Most Alpha books are available at special quantity discounts for bulk purchases for sales promotions, premiums, fund-raising, or educational use. Special books, or book excerpts, can also be created to fit specific needs.

For details, write: Special Market, Alpha Books, 375 Hudson Street, New York, NY 10014.

Contents

Foreword

In the health and fitness business, books often set the trend, they often define a generation. Often they are short-term "one-month wonders" that make a splash in the news, and a few dollars for their authors, and then (thankfully) fade from memory. Others are more enduring, defining a basic shift in how we think about health and fitness.

Sally Edwards is known for doing just this—changing how we think and act in ways that work successfully. Other authors have done the same—Ken Cooper's *Aerobics*, Dean Ornish's *Program for Reversing Heart Disease*, and Barry Sears's *The Zone* all come to mind as books that were both popular and prescient of a new wave in health and fitness. Two of Edwards's books are landmarks. In 1981, she wrote the first book about the sport of triathlon when few were participating, and today it is an Olympic sport. Another was Sally Edwards's *Heart Rate Monitor Book*, published in 1992, which essentially put the use of portable heart rate monitors on the map. Thanks to Sally, her concept of heart zones reaches everyone from the gal or guy on the treadmill next to you all the way to professional cyclists racing in the Tour de France.

In her new book, Sally and colleague Lorraine Brown take on a new challenge—the vast number of people who are regular exercisers and sometimes, like Lorraine, accomplished marathon runners and triathletes, but who will never look like Jane Fonda, or Suzanne Somers, or Bill Phillips, or any of the other gurus of the "get fit and look beautiful" school of thinking. This is not to criticize Jane and Suzanne and Bill. They got a lot of people off their backsides and into the gym; but the fact of the matter is that most people who start exercising will never look like the "after" photo one sees in the ads. Unfortunately, if the premise of exercising is to become beautiful, once people realize that they won't, then the exercise program tends to fade away. Picking up on a term probably first coined by Dr. Steven Blair of the Institute for Aerobics Research in Dallas, and countering a term used 15 years ago by Covert Bailey in his book *Fit or Fat*, this new work by Sally and Lorraine, *Fit and Fat*, addresses a more basic issue for all those who like to exercise, who want to be healthier, who want to use exercise as a tool for preventing the cardiovascular and metabolic diseases that are so common early in the twenty-first century, who want to at least feel like the "after" photo on the inside; but thanks to their choice of grandparents are never likely to be either supermodel gorgeous or, like Sally, elite athletic performers.

The text in *Fit and Fat* is straightforward, well researched, very contemporary, and linked to the concept of heart rate monitoring pioneered by Sally. But she targets her message to the mass of us "dumplings" who will never be in an ad, but who need guidance and encouragement to start and continue exercising; because it's good for us, it helps us feel better, and it's fun. Sally and Lorraine have distilled the mass of cross-talk and fitness advice into a simple and practical plan for those who hate Spandex and think exercise is for their own benefit, not a show for everyone else.

Carl Foster, Ph.D.
Professor of Exercise and Sport Science, University of Wisconsin-La Crosse, and author of *Physiological Assessment of Human Fitness*

Introduction

I am so happy you are reading this book because I believe in my heart that it will change your life. I've competed as a professional athlete all my life, winning races like the Ironman triathlon and the Western States 100 Mile Run that seem extreme to most people. But the races that inspired me to write this book were not the ones in which I broke the tape first, but rather those in which I finished dead last—behind women finishers of the Danskin Women's Triathlon Series who had only recently begun to think of themselves as athletes and who now take pride in being fit and fat.

If fat has caused you grief, made you feel badly about your body, or held you back from accomplishing your dreams, as it did for so many women I met at the back of the pack at Danskin's races, you can start changing all that today. In the pages ahead, I show you not how to get rid of your fat but how to start on the road that leads to a healthier, happier life—the road to fitness.

Recent research has shown that, contrary to a long-held myth that you can either be fit *or* fat, you actually can be both fit *and* fat. Carrying extra fat does not prevent you from possessing all the benefits of metabolic, emotional, and physical fitness.

In this book you learn about the research behind the fit-and-fat revolution. You will discover that dieting and fighting fat is a waste of time and that fitness is a much better deal. Unlike fat-loss programs, your fitness program will bring you amazing benefits in terms of your energy, self-confidence, chances of warding off chronic disease, and most important, your dreams of living a healthy, happy life.

If you have identified yourself as a fat person, you have probably ignored the athlete inside yourself. I don't mean a professional athlete or winning in competitions. I mean a person who makes fitness a daily part of his or her life. It's all about activity. As you complete the dozens of activities in this book, you will find yourself creating energy-shifting systems, managing your fat, and improving your levels of metabolic, emotional, and physical fitness.

Why should you take my word for it? I have been dedicated to helping folks get fit for the last 30 years. As a professional athlete, I have spent my life getting myself supremely fit and winning races. I've competed in some of the hardest endurance races in the world, from the Hawaiian Ironman triathlon to the Western States 100 Mile Run, from the Iditarod 100 mile snowshoe race to the Race Across America bicycle race. Throughout the years I have also run my own enterprises aimed at getting other people fit. I started the Fleet Feet chain of running stores, a state-of-the-art snowshoe manufacturing company, and a training and education company called Heart Zones. In addition, for the last 10 years I've written a series of health and fitness books.

What does a professional athlete know about fat? Well that's a good question. I hold a Master's degree in exercise physiology from the University of California and have studied, experimented with, and applied the science behind sports training and conditioning for more than 30 years. The science fascinates me—especially the latest findings from top research facilities in the world, which confirm that fitness can change your life, *no matter how much you weigh.*

In 1990, I helped found a new fitness-training program and event called the Danskin Women's Triathlon. It started that first year with 3 races with 150 participants each and has grown to a national series of 8 races with up to 4,500 participants each. I have gone to the starting line, swum a half-mile in open water, bicycled 12 miles, and crossed the finish line after a concluding 3.1 mile run/walk a hundred times, never missing a single event in the Danskin Triathlon Series. After years of racing at the front of the pack, I now finish at the back as the volunteer "final-finisher." I love it because it ensures that no woman suffers the agony of coming in last. I also love it because it's where I see the true the magic and miracle of fitness take place.

The 80,000 women who have now finished a sprint distance Danskin triathlon have inspired me. This year, as the women stood at the starting line in Seattle, Washington, I saw 4,500 women of every size, shape, age, and weight all dressed in a swimsuit or special triathlon outfit. They were nervous, tense, even downright terrified, but every single one of those women finished, and as they did, they touched the athlete inside themselves. You'll meet a lot of these women as well as other men and women like them in this book.

Fit and *Fat* presents an eight-week program to help you discover the athlete inside yourself. Each week you will learn a vital aspect of fitness, accelerate your progress toward better fitness, and participate in activities that are both fun and rewarding. You will build on what you have learned and gradually start to move more and more. Most important, you will tailor your program to your unique body, lifestyle, needs, goal, and schedule.

Here is a brief preview of your eight-week journey:

To give you a starting point, in Chapter 1, you will learn the science behind the fit-and-fat revolution and begin some simple, gentle movement.

Introduction

Then we begin our week-by-week lessons. Week 1 explains the mental shift you should make from preoccupation with fat to a dedication to fitness. You'll discover why fitness is all about your heart, and you'll conduct some basic assessments of your physical fitness.

During week 2, you'll study the language of the heart and start using your heart rate to gain insights into your emotional fitness. Simple activities with an inexpensive heart rate monitor will help you establish individual training zones to ensure you are training at the right level for you.

Week 3 reveals the flaws in the classic energy balancing equation (energy in = energy out) that drives most weight-loss programs. You'll replace that concept with insights into how real bodies function in the real world. "Energy shifting" provides a nondiet approach to eating with your metabolic, emotional, and physical health in mind.

Week 4 explains the key aspects of metabolic fitness: blood fat, sugar-insulin, and blood pressure. You will find out how physical activity, not weight loss, is the best way to become and stay metabolically healthy and dodge chronic lifestyle diseases, such as type II diabetes and cardiovascular disease.

In week 5, you'll explore the mind-body connection of emotional fitness, especially how stress can make you fat. Just like other aspects of fitness, you can train for emotional fitness by taking some assessments on which you can base emotional fitness training activities. Also in Chapter 6, you will learn more about physical fitness and how to put together your unique program, one that addresses *your* heart fitness, *your* strength, and *your* flexibility.

Week 6 will answer your questions about fat burning. You will discover that the "fat-burning zone" is a myth but that you can influence your fat burning capacity for the better through particular types of training. Believe it or not, the typical "fat-burning program" can actually *keep* you fat. By becoming more fit, you automatically become a better fat burner.

In week 7, you put all the pieces together and formulate your own plan using a process that you build step by step.

Last, in week 8, I offer some tips on how to stay motivated. You might have experienced fitness failures in the past, especially if you've ridden the diet-merry-go-round. Your new journey to fitness will succeed if you learn how to invoke the magic of motivation, set the right goals, navigate around obstacles and road blocks, boost your self-confidence, and rally your support team.

That's it in a nutshell. It will take you perhaps a dozen hours to read *Fit* and *Fat* cover to cover, and it will take you dozens more to incorporate everything you learn here into your daily life. I never make promises I can't keep, but I can make this one confidently: Give yourself eight weeks on the Fit *and* Fat program, and you'll end up giving yourself a priceless gift— a healthier, happier life.

You go, friend!
Sally Edwards
Sacramento, California

Acknowledgments

The creation of a book takes as much energy and commitment as training for and completing the Ironman Triathlon. For even the most accomplished author or the most highly trained athlete there comes a time when you feel exhausted, what competitors in endurance sports term being "caught by the man with the hammer." That's when another kind of hammer comes to the rescue, all the friends and colleagues, coaches and mentors, pick up their tools and keep hammering the nails of accomplishment. It took a lot of "hammers" to build this book:

Mike Snell, not only the biggest and boldest hammer, but our literary agent, our fellow writer, and our longtime friend and supporter.

Tracy Kelly, the woman who attains the speed of light on a keyboard.

Carl Foster, one of the best "out of the box" exercise physiologists, thinkers, and researchers in America today.

Steven Jonas, the Good Samaritan and medical doc who hammers his patients to live a long and healthy life by both example and insistence.

Covert Bailey, one of the early mentors of the Fit and Fat movement.

Glenn Gaesser, brilliant author of *Big Fat Lies*, a brilliant man.

Chris Fenn, from Scotland, one of Europe's best nutritionists.

Dan Rudd, a.k.a. "Brother Heart," who shared his expertise as one of America's foremost emotional fitness experts.

Paul Camerer, the man who constantly reminds us that fitness does not have to decline with age.

Jim Burns, the poster child of Fit *and* Fat.

Sharon Snyder, a woman who shows many who are fat that they can get fit.

Introduction

Nancy Weninger, a great proofreader and challenger of our work.

Estelle Gray, an unwavering supporter.

Kevin Brown, a true partner.

Jennifer Portnick, Anne Graham, Ann Paterson, Tina Humphreys, Kevin Brown, Louise and Richard van der Tuin, Lou Landreth, Kelly Cantrell, and *Jeanette DePatie,* the immortal folks who contributed inspirational stories of traveling the fitness highway.

CHAPTER 1

The Fit-and-Fat Revolution

Exploring What Science Tells Us About Diet and Exercise

You Can Be Fit *and* Fat

You might not think fit and fat go together, but scientists have found that they can. Now it's official: You can be fit *and* fat. Here's the story of Jennifer Portnick, who filed a Human Rights complaint against a company that said she was too fat to become one of their certified aerobics instructors. She stood up and insisted that her fatness had nothing to do with her ability to lead exercise classes, and rightly so.

Aerobics Instructor Proves You Can Be Fit *and* Fat

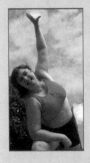

Jennifer Portnick is a 38-year-old red-haired aerobics instructor from Oakland, California, who has been working out and teaching aerobics 6 days a week for the last 15 years. You can tell she's fit by her graceful appearance and good muscular build. However, because she's 80 pounds overweight by medical standards, she qualifies as not only fat, but obese. This doesn't matter to her clients, who love her Lycra-clad, well-padded female shape and her enormous energy and vitality.

Jennifer inspires and energizes the ordinary women who come to her class to get fit. Forget her fat. She knows the extra padding doesn't harm her health because she's fit inside, and that's what really matters. However, when Jennifer applied to become a certified dance aerobics teacher with Jazzercise, Inc., the company turned her down flat because of her "appearance." They said she was too fat. She didn't embody the impossible physical dream that most fitness instructors display, so she didn't meet their standards. Fat instructors, they argued, could not be fit.

When Jennifer got the letter from Jazzercise telling her that she needed to display a "more fit appearance" and that a Jazzercise teacher must look "leaner than the public," she was devastated. "I felt that this was not a valid judgment of me. I only ask that I be judged on my merits," she says. After all, her own instructor, impressed with Jennifer's stamina and ability in class, had urged her to apply.

Fortunately, Jennifer lives in the city of San Francisco, where a recently implemented law prohibits discrimination on the basis of weight and height. The law says that if a person can do the job, weight shouldn't matter. "Being an aerobics instructor is a skill-based job, and I had all the skills," Jennifer recalls. So in September 2001, she filed a complaint with the city's Human Rights Commission. Meanwhile, Jennifer earned certification through the Aerobics and Fitness Association of America and now teaches high-energy, low-impact classes in a health studio in the vibrant San Francisco South of Market district. "I want to offer people the opportunity to feel good about their bodies, whatever the size and shape may be," she says.

In April 2002, Jazzercise, Inc., and Jennifer reached a mutually acceptable agreement after legal mediation and settled the claim without the Human Rights Commission rendering a judgment. The company had changed its mind and accepted that a person can be both fit and fat. "Empirically I am healthy," she insists. "All my vitals are normal, my blood pressure is normal, my blood sugar is normal. I am healthy." She challenged the establishment and won.

How about you? Where would you place yourself on the Fit *and* Fat continuum? Are you fat? If you are, are you fit? If you think you are fat by your doctor's standards, your standards, or anybody else's, or if fat has affected your life in any way, this book is for you. Have you suffered because of fat—fat as a condition, fat as an issue, fat prejudice, or fat simply as an debilitating illusion of mind and a means of self-denial? If so, I wrote this book for you because I believe this eight-week Heart Zones program can put a stop to all that suffering and free you from all the "fat" weighing so heavily on your body and soul. I do not promise you that you will get slim. Nor do I expect you to compete in a triathlon in two months. But I can guarantee this: If you embark on this program, you will find yourself in the good company of people like those who've worked out with Jennifer—more fit, a little less fat, happier, and definitely healthier.

Modern media, the diet industry, advertising, and social prejudices against fat have created a myth that you must be slim to be healthy and happy. This makes me angry because not only does it cause a lot of emotional damage, but it also distracts us from the real issue: that *fitness*, not fatness, deserves our full attention if we want to enjoy a long, healthy life.

My aim is to empower you to stop fighting fat and to start fighting for your fitness and your health instead. To do so, you'll need both the facts revealed in recent scientific studies and a fitness program based on those facts. Armed with those tools, you can begin climbing out of the big fat hole you may have fallen into while you were trying to get thin through dieting. Forgive me for repeating myself, but this program is not designed to make you skinny. Skinny is for fashion magazine models and television sitcom actresses. Don't think thin—think fit.

Inside every person is an athlete. Imagine a huge SUV with a bumper sticker that reads, "Inside me is a racing car." No matter how big and ungainly it looks, the SUV really does have a powerful turbo engine under its hood. It might not win the Indianapolis 500, but it will go around the track 200 times at a pretty good clip.

Have you been hoodwinked into thinking only about the extra fat you carry on the outside, only to ignore what's going on "under the hood"? Your engine inside gives you energy, provides the motivation to do the things you want to do in life, and powers you to go out and do them. I'm talking about your inner power and essence, what's in both your physical and your emotional heart. Fat itself cannot hold you back unless you let it. When you develop a fit heart, nothing can stop you.

If you have been starving yourself for years, in terms of both how you treat your blood-pumping heart and how you feel about yourself, you might have a sick engine under your hood, a sticky engine with parts that don't run smoothly. In some places, the parts might have partly seized up, while others might not be working at all. If you listened to it carefully, you could hear it struggling, especially when you tax it with extra effort. All that time you spent concentrating on the bodywork, the fancy wheels, and the paint job didn't create a lean machine.

So why don't you take time now to look under the hood and consider what your inner engine needs to get stronger and stop holding you back in life?

Remember the powerful engine inside the big SUV. I want you to reconnect with that engine. I want you to realize the power of that racing car within and put it to good use in your life. I want you to find that athlete inside!

Are you muttering, "No, that's not for me. I can't be an athlete. Athletes wear skinny Lycra outfits and race around running tracks like Greyhounds. I'm just an old St. Bernard"? Yes, that might be true if we were talking about the Olympics, but such high-performance athletes represent an extreme condition of genetic heritage and a lifetime of dedication that most of us will never approach. What I mean by "athlete" is a person who respects his or her racing engine and uses it to power their way to whatever goals that person wants to achieve in life. All it takes is an understanding and an appreciation of your body as a partner in life rather than as an obstacle that gets in the way and has to be punished with diets.

Fat Trap: The Dangers of Fat Loss

Weight loss can actually be harmful to your health. In his pivotal and groundbreaking book *Big Fat Lies*,[1] Glenn Gaesser, Ph.D., a professor at the University of Virginia, includes a chapter entitled "Diet and Die" that warns of the dangers posed by weight loss and weight fluctuations. According to Gaesser, between 1983 and 1993, 15 published studies demonstrated that weight loss *increases* the risk of premature death, sometimes by up to 260 percent. In the same time period, only three published articles demonstrated the health benefits of weight loss (in one, a weight loss of 1 pound bought you an 11-hour extension to your life).

Cherish your body with healthy and nutritious food, good fun, frequent physical activity, and an ongoing healthy lifestyle, and you will unleash the power to set goals and achieve them, releasing yourself from the fear of fat that has been holding you back.

You Don't Have to Be Thin to Be Fit

If your genetic heritage and metabolism make you susceptible to gaining fat very easily, don't feel bad. You could be one of evolution's triumphs. In evolutionary terms, the people who fared the best through times of sporadic food supply were the ones whose bodies made the most efficient use of energy and stored away as much as possible for later use. Scientists now know we evolved to succeed in an environment when food supply was unreliable and the physical demands of life were high. Imagine yourself in this environment, pitted for survival against that skinny fashion model with no apparent body fat. Who would live longer? To paraphrase Darwin, it all comes down to "survival of the fattest (and fittest)."

But you may be thinking, "I don't want to be the fattest guy in the cave. I need to go on a diet and get some of the weight off before I can survive a stroll through the jungle." That's where you are wrong—dead wrong. Fitness and thinness are not the same thing. They are not connected. Sure, you probably know a lot of fat and unfit people, and they may have gotten fat because they got unfit. But it is possible for a person to be fat and fit. Fitness correlates to how well your engine is running, not to streamlined fenders or narrow tires.

Think about that for a moment, because it's really important. Do you perceive all slender people as fit? Do you define all fat people as unfit? If so, you've fallen for a big, fat lie. In terms of fitness, what you see is not necessarily what you get. Look inside—evaluate the engine before you pass judgment.

The Athlete Inside: Lorraine Brown's Story

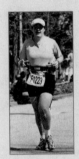

I'm glad I looked inside Lorraine Brown. And she's glad she looked inside herself. A 30-year-old overweight and unfit woman when I first met her, Lorraine eventually found the athlete hiding inside. I'll let her tell her own story in her own words:

My first athletic experience in adult life was taking part in my first triathlon. My previous athletic experience had been the harrowing sport sessions as a child at school, where I was ridiculed for always coming in last. I never wanted to go there again. And I didn't, until one day my friend, Sally, persuaded me to do my first triathlon. In fact, all it took was for her to say, "Lorraine, I think you can do it." Nobody had ever said that to me before. With that simple sentence, Sally had reached inside and touched a raw nerve. Of course, I would have liked to have been more physically able at school, to be able to run the cross-country course like the others. After all, it seemed like they were having fun, but I just couldn't run the course.

Six months after my conversation with Sally, I found myself traveling to Disney World in Florida all the way from Scotland to do my first triathlon. I had gotten married the day before, so my husband and I made it our honeymoon. What an incredible week for me!

The experience was a tremendous one, and when I finished, I felt so proud of what I had done. But it was a little sign that nearly made me cry: the one directing the participants in the race to the starting area. It read, "Athletes, this way."

At first glance, I didn't get it. I would have been less surprised to see one that read, "Fat girls, this way." Then I heard my inner voice say, "That's me. I'm an athlete."

It was the first time in my life that I had found and felt my athlete inside. She had been there my whole life, but I discovered her only that morning on the way to the starting line of my first triathlon.

Why Are We All Getting Fatter?

Every day, the media reports on how fat Americans are getting. Our country now tops the world in terms of girth as well as trade. A visitor from another planet might find it ironic that we seem to be drowning ourselves in the fat of our own affluence. The media, the medical community, and the health industry all place the blame for this trend firmly on each individual consumer's lack of restraint at the dinner table. Although it's true that each of us does choose every day what we put in our mouths, it's not entirely true that consumers deserve all the blame for getting so fat. We live in a society that puts huge demands and pressures on us, influences the amount and quality of what we eat, and limits our opportunities and choices within certain boundaries. An understanding of this environment will do a lot more than another round of guilt analysis to get us on the path to fitness. Such an understanding will help us regain individual power over our lives, overcome feelings of helplessness about making crucial changes, and start making those changes.

Researchers who have examined the reasons for the expansion of Americans' midsections have offered these possible explanations:

- We're eating more today than we did in the past. We expend the same amount of energy, so our weight has naturally gone up.
- We're eating the same as we used to, but we expend less energy, resulting in more stored fat.
- We actually eat less today, but our energy expenditure has dropped so much that we store excess energy as fat.

In fact, when scientists surveyed eating patterns in many different western countries, they found that caloric intake has not actually increased over the last 25 years or so.[2] At the same time, our intake of calories derived from fat has also diminished. These findings argue that physical activity must play a key role in the equation. Otherwise, how could we be eating less but getting fatter? Scientists have concluded that, in general, the rise in obesity stems from a lack of physical activity. The researchers analyzing the extent to which our present-day lives differ from those of the past estimate that we have denied ourselves as much as 800 calories of daily physical activity by relying on car transport, energy-saving devices, and performing less and less manual labor.[3] That means that our ancestors may have used up to 800 calories a day more than us tracking down their food, carrying water, scrubbing clothes, fetching firewood, walking to school, or riding a bike to the shops.

Today we live in a world crammed with devices designed to save us effort, from power windows in our cars to automatically opening doors at the supermarket. And everywhere we turn, we see tasty food readily available in mere minutes. All this has convinced scientists that we have fashioned an environment for ourselves in which it's inevitable that we'll get fat. We're programmed to like tasty food, and our bodies can't effectively regulate our weight when we don't get enough exercise. As Claude Bouchard, an internationally respected authority on obesity from the Pennington Biomedical Research Center at Louisiana State University, says in the introduction to the book *Physical Activity and Obesity*, "[Human] biological systems cannot cope well in an environment in which palatable foods are abundant and energy expenditure of activity is low. It seems to be extremely difficult for many of us to regulate food and caloric intake to be in balance at low levels of daily energy expenditure."[4]

In our modern world, Bouchard concludes that inadequate exercise prevents our bodies from functioning normally. Instead of regulating their weight in a natural way, many people can maintain a normal weight only by constantly restricting calories. They diet. And that doesn't work in the long run. In the long run, only proper exercise will allow your body to do its job normally.

Fat Trap: Are My Genes Making Me Fat?

A lot of talk recently has focused on the genetics of fatness. You may have heard that scientists have discovered a fat gene. They've even been able to breed specially fat mice. You might even have heard about the gene for leptin, a substance that tells the brain you've had enough to eat. When people lack the gene that governs leptin production, they get fat. All this is true.

In fact, researchers have identified at least 75 genes that play a role in obesity. However, we can't chalk up the recent rise in overweight and obesity in the United States to altered genes. It's just not biologically possible for our genetic makeups to change over a mere 25 years. Such a change takes much longer.

More clues to how our genetics affect weight and fatness have come from studies of people who move from one lifestyle to another, populations like Pima Indians and Africans moving to the United States and adopting a different lifestyle, usually one characterized by more food and less exercise. Researchers have found that, yes, certain genetic factors do make us susceptible to getting fat, but we get fat only when we put ourselves in an environment where that can happen. The key triggers for the expression of "fat" genes? A fat-rich, plentiful food supply and a couch-potato lifestyle.

The Big, Fat Lie

For years, diet experts have insisted that we focus on fat, fat-burning, fat-free foods, good fat, bad fat, fat, fat, fat. Fat's bad. Get rid of it. What's the first thing a physician will say to a fat person in his office, no matter what his or her complaint? "Well, you're just too darned fat," as if getting rid of fat would cure all health disorders. It's not surprising that many fat people dread visiting a medical professional and, therefore, don't get the level of medical care they deserve. These people have been badly advised and poorly served by the medical profession.

Here's a simple truth: *Fat is a symptom of obesity, not the cause.* The definition of obesity relates to its physical characteristics: the percentage of fat you carry relative to your body weight. I am sure in years to come we will look back in astonishment at such a simplistic view. It's like looking at a case of the measles and calling it "skin lesions," when we really know it is a respiratory infection caused by the measles virus. The spots are just a symptom. Defining obesity by one of the physical symptoms ignores what goes on inside the body. In truth, obesity is the condition by which the complex mechanisms of appetite and satiety (how you feel) and how the body converts the food you eat into energy (metabolism) have, quite simply, become messed up. Our body's weight-regulatory system has gone haywire, usually because of metabolic, physical, or emotional abuse of the body.

An all too common example of metabolic abuse is serial dieting. The body fights periodic starvation by making key metabolic changes that make sure you gain the weight back when you eat even a normal, healthy diet. The metabolism can become so dysfunctional that the body can function only by grabbing and storing all the energy that comes its way.

We commit a form of physical abuse when we don't perform the basic physical activity we need to stay healthy. Amazingly, we readily accept that our Springer Spaniel needs exercise to stay healthy, but we don't recognize the same for ourselves.

Finally, emotional overload, such as stress, can throw the body out of sync and disrupt its weight-regulating system.

If you are fatter than you think you should be or you have gained a lot of fat, take a close look at those three factors: your metabolic, physical, and emotional health. You might find that you've neglected one or more of these key aspects of health. Your sense of fatness might derive from underlying problems with any or all of them.

Fat Trap: Obesity as a Disease

Every day, we hear obesity described as "an epidemic of fat people." Imagine how that makes a fat person feel. Like a germ. Yes, in the United States, excess fat is now officially a disease, thanks to the media running wild with the idea of fat as a disease. It's such a shame because the negative perception is more harmful than all the fat cells in the world. Many well-intentioned doctors have lobbied to remove the stigma of obesity as a character flaw or personal failing. But the fat-loss industry, including pharmaceutical companies and weight-loss treatment programs, embraced this so they could justify the sales of drugs and remedies, and clear the way for medical insurance claims and tax deductions. However, the truth about obesity has gotten lost in all the furor: Leading obesity experts now see obesity as the condition of a dysfunctional weight-regulating system, not as a behavioral or mental illness.

If you have always been a little fat, yet you've cared for the three basic aspects of your health, then consider your specific biological makeup, your inherited genetics, and your individual physiology. Our genetic heritage extends not only to whether we possess our mother's eyes or our father's chin, but to the nature of our metabolism and to how we respond to physical fitness training. Our individual biological makeup even means that each one of us differs in terms of how our internal biochemical processes work, including everything from adrenaline production, digestive processes, fat metabolism, insulin, and regulation and fluctuations in sex hormones.

Once you understand your biological makeup, you can stop fretting over the fact that you didn't inherit the physique of a teenage fashion model. Perhaps you should stop trying to be something you can't be. After all, you'd never buy a St. Bernard dog and think, "Ah, well, if I starve Bernie enough, maybe I can make him look like a Greyhound. Greyhounds are so fashionable this year, and I want a fashionable dog." No, you treasure all your big, lovable St. Bernard's qualities. You like big dogs. Why not like your big self? We humans come in all shapes and sizes, so why should we all want to look like those skinny people on *Ally McBeal*?

The Amazon Woman: Anne's Story

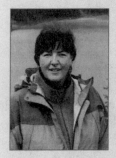

My friend Anne Graham learned to love her body— and what it can do—when she accepted her biological makeup and started thinking of herself as an Amazon woman. Here's her story:

One of the dreaded put-downs in my family was to be called a "wimp." We were a raucous, rowdy, active family of five kids, all of us hard players and hardy eaters. We biked, went cross-country skiing, swam, and roamed the countryside as a way of life in rural Wisconsin. Seventy-mile bike rides were not uncommon in my teens. It was a virtue to be big, healthy, strong, and capable. When I moved into my teen years, these same qualities made me feel lumbering, unfeminine, and horsey, like a Clydesdale horse. While people didn't usually think of me as fat, I made that translation in my head. I could be described as stocky, solid, or big-boned. And the height-weight charts unequivocally said I was overweight (I still am). But I took pride in being an Amazon, a strong and physically capable woman. Size isn't everything, and I sure got around and had some fun!

Having held mostly sedentary jobs during much of my adult life, I had gotten away from fitness for large chunks of time. As I got deeper into middle age, my strength seemed to fade during those months or years when I was out of shape. I was alarmed to be getting bigger and losing my ability to pick up and do harder things, such as backpacking. I became less interested in participating with friends on an outing that was physically difficult, such as a hike with much elevation gain (common here in the Pacific Northwest). Previously, I had felt mostly okay about being bigger than most women because my strength had always made up for it. Then one day I was on a back-country ski trip when it hit me: I was just another overweight and very out-of-shape woman. I had to make up my mind about what path to follow into later middle age and beyond.

I decided that it wasn't too late. I could reclaim myself by finding the fun in physical activity that I had loved as a kid. It wasn't too late to stop my body's slide into fat and flab and turn it around to become a fit, energetic, strong Amazon again.

But it is such a catch-22! When you are out of shape, you don't want to exercise because it is too hard; then not exercising makes you more and more out of shape! To find a motivation to get started, I used fun and variety in my workouts to lure me beyond the discomforts of being heavy with no strength, having a very large bust, and being in poor cardiovascular condition. I also set myself a goal: to do a triathlon. I wasn't too hard on myself if I didn't feel like pushing it some days, but I still got out and did something. Exercising got easier and more addictive once some of the flab turned to muscle. I was hooked!

And I reaped my rewards: I lost a little weight and got much stronger. The scale doesn't report a much lower number, and I doubt I will ever be thin because it isn't in my nature or in my genes. I am still the hardy eater I was as a kid. But I see my body's changes and relish them: a smaller bust and waist; serious, muscular legs and arms; and the energy and eagerness to tackle physically challenging activities. I keep up with people decades younger, and I feel fully alive. I am still a big woman, but an Amazon, not a fat lady.

Sometimes we talk ourselves into a corner, saying, "Well, even though I was born with this body type, it can't be natural for me to be like this because this is an unhealthy state. How can it be okay that I was born unhealthy?" Such thinking reflects one of the problems the fat-free movement has created for us: We have forgotten why we have fat and what it does for us. We've forgotten that it is natural for some of us to be fatter than others, even if it places us outside the recommended weight for our height (an unreliable recommendation, as we will see).

Fat is a natural thing, an essential ingredient in a healthy body. It's not just a nasty lump of inanimate matter. Most fat works for us in life-sustaining ways, protecting our vital organs, insulating us, and storing energy so we can function without constant eating. Some special types of fat cells perform absolutely crucial tasks, such as dealing with toxins in the body and maintaining a healthy hormonal balance. We need fat, and we need to store extra fat. It's also natural for us to gain more fat as we age. It's natural for some of us to carry more fat than others. But it's *not* natural for us to be unfit. Our bodies require physical activity as much as they require air, water, and fuel. Without it, we die. And this brings us to the crux of the matter: We have become stuck in the mind-set that being fat makes us sick, when, in truth, being unfit makes us sick. When we grasp that fact, we begin to realize that fat loss as a solution to health problems is just a fiction.

Fitness Versus Fatness

Let's explore what we mean by fitness and fatness. Fitness measures how healthy you are, how functionally able you are to carry out your daily life. Fatness measures the amount of padding you carry—how big your fenders are, not the strength of the inner engine that gives you the power to do things in life.

Fitness might mean one thing to a professional basketball player and another to a young woman with a family and career, but basically it all boils down to being healthy and in good condition, with the energy and optimism to tackle your dreams and goals. To attain fitness, you must consider the three components we mentioned before:

- **Metabolic fitness.** Your blood pressure, glucose sensitivity, and blood chemistry.
- **Physical fitness.** Your cardiovascular fitness (heart and circulatory system), muscular strength, and flexibility.
- **Emotional fitness.** Your ability to access and balance your feelings.

Keeping this list in mind, try answering these three questions:

- Can people display healthy blood chemistry and a healthy metabolism even if they are fat?
- Can people possess a strong, healthy heart and be physically strong and flexible even if they are fat?
- Can people maintain emotional balance even if they are fat?

The answer to all three questions? A resounding "Yes." It's that simple. Fatness does not prevent fitness. The amount of fat you carry around represents but one aspect of your health and fitness, and not necessarily a terribly relevant one at that. In contrast, physical, emotional, and metabolic fitness provide the keys to a healthy and long life. Being thin will never guarantee you a long life. Being fit in terms of cardiovascular, metabolic, and blood chemistry health will. The proof depends on scientific research, not on myths and fads.

"USA Scientist: Fat Can Be Healthy"

Did you see that headline on the CNN news service on July 18, 2001?[5] American researcher Steven Blair had sparked controversy at a meeting of the Association for the Study of Obesity in London by saying that body fat can be healthy. Results from the studies at Blair's institute, The Cooper Institute, on obesity and risk of death showed that previous research had missed the crucial link between fitness and health. "The focus is all wrong," claimed Blair, Ph.D., who continued to say, "It is fitness that is the key." In fact, he even went on to report quite simply that "fat people who exercise are at no greater risk from disease than their thinner, lazier counterparts."

Our obsession with weight and weight loss has misled us to blame fat and fatness as the root of all illness. In fact, according to Blair, nothing can improve your health risks more than fitness.

Not surprisingly, Blair's claims ignited some criticism. For instance, the spokesperson for the International Obesity Taskforce said that the findings trivialized the debate.[6] Back in 1998, Dr. Andrew Prentice, currently at the MRC International Nutrition Group, Public Health Unit at the London School of Hygiene and Tropical Medicine, had set the stage for this reaction by insisting, "I think it's quite dangerous to suggest that it is okay to be fat, and really it is fitness that counts. We know this is not the case."[7] In recent years, however, the evidence supporting Blair's claim that fitness confers a lower risk of disease and mortality, independent of fatness, has been pouring in:

- A study published in the October 1999 issue of the *Journal of the American Medical Association* found that overweight men *who exercised* had death rates, by any cause, only slightly higher than those of fit men of normal weight and twice as low as those of normal weight men who were unfit.[8]

- An observational study carried out by three researchers, Chong Do Lee, Steven Blair, and Andrew Jackson, at the Cooper Institute for Aerobics Research in Dallas, Texas,[9] demonstrated that it's fitness, not fatness, that really counts when it comes to longevity. In their observational study of 22,000 men, they found that death rates doubled for unfit men. Interestingly, obese men had no greater risk of dying than men of normal weight, as long as they were fit. The researchers concluded that being fit reduces the health risk of being obese.

- A study of 17,000 men in the Harvard Alumni Health Study[10] found that mortality was lower for each category of increasing fatness when the men were fit.

- Researchers Steven Blair and Suzanne Brodney at the Cooper Institute in Dallas, Texas, conducted a review of all studies that had been done up to 1999, examining over 700 scientific articles. They concluded that regular physical activity clearly mitigates many of the health risks associated with being overweight or obese, and that fat people who are fit have lower death rates than normal-weight individuals who are not fit.[11]

The American College of Sports Medicine (ACSM) together with the U.S. National Institutes of Health and National Heart, Lung, and Blood Institute (NIH) commissioned reviews of all this new evidence, hoping they could prepare consensus statements concerning the benefits of physical activity for overweight people. The review concluded that the recent scientific research shows the following:

- Overweight and obese individuals who are active and fit have lower rates of disease and death than overweight and obese individuals who are inactive and unfit.

- Overweight or obese individuals who are active and fit are less likely to develop obesity-related chronic diseases and suffer early death than normal-weight persons who lead sedentary lives.

- Inactivity and low cardiorespiratory fitness are as important as overweight or obesity as predictors of mortality, at least in men.[12, 13]

Taking the *or* Out of the "Fit or Fat"

The notion that fatness indicates bad health and risk of disease may have existed long before Covert Bailey came on the scene, but he certainly popularized it. In the early 1970s, Bailey, a marketing genius, published a best-selling book titled *Fit or Fat* that, more than anything else, popularized the view that you have two choices in life: You can either be fit or you can be fat. His message found a ready audience, and his books went on to sell more than four million copies. To his credit, Bailey tried to help his readers improve their health through exercise, and many have benefited from his work. But, as science has shown, Bailey had it wrong. You *can* be fit *and* fat.

Once Bailey coined the phrase "fit *or* fat," the medical profession, the diet industry, the fashion industry, and advertisers all trumpeted it. Why did millions of people buy into it? The answer traces its roots all the way back to the turn of the century, when life insurance companies such as the Metropolitan Life Insurance Company began looking for ways to minimize their liability and maximize their profits by screening people before they issued policies. In 1942 and 1943, Metropolitan's efforts resulted in the modern-day height-weight tables, which clearly reflected the idea that thinner is better.

The height-weight data reflected a positive relationship between weight and mortality: The more people weighed, the sooner they died. Then the search started for the link between obesity and disease. Subsequent studies concluded that obesity causes many of the serious health conditions that lower our life expectancy. These killers include hypertension, type II diabetes, coronary heart disease, gallbladder disease, certain cancers, increased blood fats (triglycerides), stroke, osteoarthritis, and sleep apnea.

As it turns out, however, all this failed to include the role of fitness as an independent variable. For example, in one study you would have found a positive relationship between fatness and mortality if you just lumped all fat men into one group. Only when you separated two groups from the population (the fat and unfit men versus the fat and fit men) could you see the truth. The fat *and* fit men died no sooner than the thin and unfit men. Fitness obviously led to longer life spans. A third group, the fat and unfit men, suffered triple the death rates of the thinner men, a fact that lowered the overall average. The bottom line? Fit people, be they fat or thin, live longer than unfit people. That statement may strike you as obvious today, but it took us decades to bring it to light.

You Can Be Fit, Fat, and Healthy

What about the research into obesity that shows that fat people are more likely to die of heart disease, diabetes, cancer, and just about everything else? Again, in the past, most researchers did not look at the fitness of the people they measured; instead, they looked at only their fatness. To date, not one single study has shown a *causal* relationship between being fat and dying early—only strong *associations*, such as that *some* people with extra fat also *happen* to experience a higher incidence of some diseases. Because about half the overweight and obese people in any one study are unfit, these studies do not offer much proof that extra fat causes specific health risks.

Some fat and unfit people, those who live a sedentary lifestyle, share a common denominator linked to disease: lack of fitness, not an overabundance of fatness. Researchers have been pointing the finger of guilt at the wrong culprit, singling out fat as the problem when, in fact, poor fitness contributes much more to health problems. If you want to arrest the right culprits, put the handcuffs on the absence of physical, emotional, and metabolic fitness.

The latest research on longevity and fitness and fatness has looked not only at *when* people die, but also *why*. These studies have examined the relationships between fitness and the specific diseases that we once thought resulted from obesity, including hypertension, type II diabetes, and coronary heart disease. In all cases, the risk of dying from one of these diseases correlates more strongly to lack of fitness than to fatness, per se. When people are fit, they have a lower incidence of a number of diseases, compared to unfit people. Now it seems clear that fitness protects against coronary heart disease, hypertension, type II diabetes, Alzheimer's disease, and even, to some degree, cancer.[14] Fitness even serves as a much better predictor of the risk of dying of cardiovascular disease than family history or smoking.

Get Fitter, Live Longer

Great news continues to pour in about fitness and the benefits it bestows. Not only does fitness help free you from life-shortening disease, but it can extend your life expectancy, too. But don't just take my word for it.

A new study published in the *New England Journal of Medicine*[15] details new evidence regarding the relationship between fitness and survival. In it, researchers examined more than 6,000 male patients referred to a clinical exercise-testing laboratory and then followed the group for 6 years. They found that the peak exercise capacity (a measure of their fitness) achieved by a person during the exercise test was the best predictor of the risk of death, whether the individual suffered from cardiovascular disease or not. For both groups, the fittest, regardless of their fatness, had a four times lower risk of dying compared to the unfit groups. As with earlier studies, fatness accompanied by fitness did not figure significantly in risk of death. Fitness extends life.

I shouldn't need to repeat it at this point: The fitter you are, the longer you can live.

Move Above the Line

So there you have it. Don't expect great health benefits from fat loss and dieting. Yes, you may have a problem losing weight, but the problem is not your fatness. Fatness is merely a symptom, not a cause. And fat loss cures nothing and can actually do a lot of harm. Forget "fit *or* fat." It's a myth. Remember "fit *and* fat." It's the truth. Fitness protects against the many diseases and prolongs life. When you are fit, you can be just as healthy as your thin cousins. Now, armed with what you've learned so far, where would you place yourself in The Fit *and* Fat Matrix?

This matrix includes four different quadrants representing various combinations of fitness and fatness.

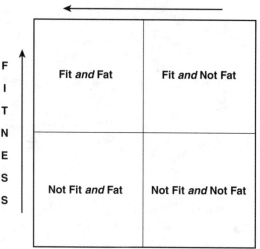

The Fit and Fat Matrix.

This one diagram helps you figure out where you are today and where you might want to go tomorrow. We know from all we have learned so far that the quadrants with the least risk of death, lowest disease rates, and best quality of life are the top two above the line (Fit *and* Fat or Fit *and* Not Fat). If you want to enjoy a long and healthy life, you need to live above the line. Now what surprises most people is that the two top quadrants provide the *same* benefits in terms of health and longevity. It doesn't matter for your health whether you sit in the Fit *and* Fat (top-left) quadrant or the Fit *and* Not Fat quadrant (top-right). Actually, the top two quadrants should be merged, as in the following figure. If at the moment you reside below the line in either of the lower two quadrants, you obviously want to move above the line. How do you do that? Well, there's only one escape route: You need to get fit. Becoming less fat will allow you to move only sideways on the quadrant, not to a higher level of health and well-being.

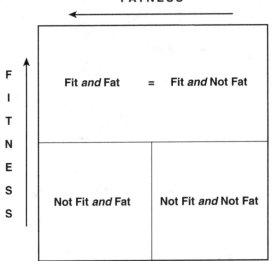

The Modified Fit and Fat Matrix.

Moving Above the Line: Lorraine Brown's Story

Read Lorraine's story of how she moved from the Not Fit and Fat quadrant to the Fit and Fat quadrant:

I struggled to be thin my whole life. I was an 11-pound baby, a fat toddler, and a fat schoolchild. As soon as I was old enough to be compared to the height-weight tables, I was sent off to the hospital dietitian to get my first diet. I was only six years old.

After a bad start in terms of weight and suffering from fat, I didn't do too badly. I did try lots of diets in my teens and, after years of torturing myself, realized that it just wasn't worth it and that I had better just accept it and get on with life rather than let it be an obsession that could ruin my life. I learned to live with my body, enjoy my physical appearance, and do things it did well, such as mountain climbing and hiking. I learned to eat healthfully, to feel well, and to enjoy life.

Then, in my late 20s, during one of those periods of reviewing my life to make sure I was on the right track, I realized I really wanted to go and climb a big mountain. I did some research, chose my mountain, and got all the information I could about Mount Logan in Alaska.

I wanted to climb the mountain, but I knew that I would probably never pass the selection process and be accepted on the expedition team. I probably wasn't fit enough to keep up, and, well, I was just too fat! This realization caught me off guard. It had been years since I had noticed that my fat had stopped me from doing something I really wanted to do. Now this obstacle suddenly reminded me of my fundamental inadequacy in life: At heart, I was just a "good-for-nothing fat person."

I went through a familiar round of "beating myself up" and feeling helpless. What could I do? Diets don't work, I knew that, so forget about that. I was already practicing healthy eating, and I had an active lifestyle.

Then I came upon the heart rate monitor. It was a gift for my birthday. I'd told my boyfriend (now husband!) that I wanted one because I'd seen other people at the gym using one and it looked interesting. When I started using it, the numbers fascinated me. "Look, that's my heart beating!" Then I got a bit more curious: What did the numbers actually mean?

My curiosity took me to the Internet, where I learned about Sally Edwards's Heart Zones Training and how to interpret the language of the heart. I realized that it was my fitness that was letting me down, not my excess fatness. I determined to get fit and not worry about the fat for a while. When I began focusing on the fitness side of life rather than on the fat, it suddenly started to work. True, I lost some weight (not enough to get out of the "obese" category on the medical height-weight charts), but what I gained was more exciting than I ever could have imagined. I discovered that I could be an athlete and do things I'd only ever imagined a person could do. That year I completed a four-day mountain bike challenge across Scotland and raced in and finished my first triathlon. This year I ran my first marathon. I'm no longer terrified of the fat gain associated with pregnancy. Who knows where it will end? One day I am going to complete an Ironman triathlon competition. I know that. What I can't believe is that it took me 30 years to realize what I could do if I would only stop letting fat hold me back. I hope it's another 30 before I discover how far I can go.

Who Wants to Be Fat and Fit?

Most of us want to be thin. Society wants us to be thin. Markets and the media want us to be thin. But deep down, do you want what others demand, or would you prefer the good health that will give you a better and longer life? We've been led into thinking that thinness will win both fashionable good looks and a good life. However, the scientific evidence says, "Hogwash!" Long life comes from health, not thinness. And health comes from fitness, not lack of fatness. So what do you really want? I honestly believe that most of us place a long, healthy life first and foremost, and fashion way down the list. That's why you should make getting fit your number-one priority. Once you gain the health benefits of fitness, natural weight loss becomes easier, almost automatic. When it comes to losing weight, living "above the line" gives you a huge advantage over those who languish "below the line."

If you still need convincing, consider this one last reason why you should focus on getting yourself fit, even if you are fat. If you've tried to get thin, you've undoubtedly waged a long, hard battle. In truth, only 5 to 10 percent of people who successfully lose weight by dieting keep it off for the first year— not a very encouraging statistic. Science now knows that the best way to lose weight and keep it off is to take it off over a relatively long period of time. In Chapter 4, we'll explore the complicated mechanisms that produce this phenomenon, but for now just bear in mind that slow, steady weight loss works much better than any quick fix.

If you focus on long-term physical, emotional, and metabolic fitness, your health will improve. It's all a matter of basic human physiology, the way the body works, and how your biological makeup responds. I promise you that if you follow the Fit *and* Fat program, you will get the health benefits you seek. You can achieve really big fitness gains in just eight weeks and hugely significant changes over eight months. You'll find the benefits and changes you make in your life far greater than those obtained by decreased fatness. No matter what your current body weight is, you'll enjoy a better self-image, improved self-confidence, and increased mobility. And you will know deep down that you are doing something for your own health—for you, and not other people. Under the hood, your engine will start firing on all eight cylinders.

You can be fit *and* fat. You may have extra body weight, but if you participate in a physically, emotionally, and metabolically sound program, you can attain a healthy body free from the risks of the diseases once so commonly linked to obesity, from coronary heart disease to adult-onset diabetes. People who are fit, even if they are fat, can expect to live longer than similarly fat people who are not fit—and even longer than lean people who are not fit. And you can much more easily achieve fitness than leanness. Won't you join me on the journey to fitness? You'll find the first step amazingly easy.

The First Step: The 800-Calorie Rule

In our modern society, a typical individual expends up to 800 fewer calories per day compared to our ancestors. This is not simply a matter of balancing the energy equation. After all, we typically not only do less than our grandparents did, but we eat less, too. The lack of up to 800 calories of work per day means we don't get the basic level of physical activity we need to function well. Add to this predicament a plentiful supply of tasty food, a high-stress lifestyle, and we can easily find ourselves plagued with poor metabolic, physical, and even emotional health. The 800-calorie rule is a first step towards correcting this situation.

To reclaim some of your lost vital physical activity, make a list of all the opportunities where you could increase your physical activity, even slightly. These might include taking the stairs rather than the elevator up to the office, parking your car at the far end of the parking lot, buying a fitness toy to play with during telephone conversations in the office, or getting off the bus one stop early. I'm not suggesting that you start washing the clothes by hand or fetching water from the creek, but I am saying that even small energy-expending investments will get you back some of the daily physical activity that can keep you healthy. Start today. When you have made your list of activities, start trying them out. Can you make some of them daily habits? Here's what Lorraine decided to try:

- I will ride my bike to work when the temperature is above freezing.
- I will take the stairs and not the elevator except when I'm carrying heavy items in two hands.
- I will scrub the kitchen carpet by hand instead of paying a man with a machine to do it.
- I will ride my bike to the gym rather than go by car.
- I will wash up more by hand and use the dishwasher less.
- I will fetch the groceries from the store by bike.
- I will take a walk around the grounds of our company at lunchtime.
- I will cycle into town on Saturday rather than take the train.

Now think what you can do. Make a list of activities that you can incorporate into your daily life that will increase your energy expenditure. Pin your list up in a prominent place to remind yourself to follow the "800-Calorie Rule."

The Eight-Week Fit *and* Fat Training Program

I've designed a fitness program that could help you change your life. I guarantee that if you follow it, your life quality will improve in metabolic, physical, and emotional ways. It's not a game of calorie counting, starvation, and guilt, but an empowering way to learn how to give your body what it needs in terms of physical activity, energy, and care. It focuses on fitness, not fatness, and it will enable you to reach your full potential in life, regardless of the amount of extra fat you carry on your body.

I want you to remember that you may not lose all of the fat that you dream about losing—at least, not in the short run. But I also want you to know that a long-term commitment will create all the positive changes that will ease off plenty of pounds. You will burn lots of stored body fat on this program, and you'll do it in surprisingly simple ways. I'll show you exactly how to do it, how to build that wonderful body into a metabolically efficient and fat-burning engine.

In the pages ahead, you will learn about energy—how to fuel your body and how to energize it to do what you want it to do. You will discover dozens of fat traps, the common mistakes you can so easily make with fat. You'll also meet lots of real fit and fat people, like Lorraine and Anne, who have changed their lives with fitness. Rather than preoccupying yourself with fat loss, fat quantity, and fat burning, or with weight or body composition, you'll concentrate on metabolic, physical, and emotional fitness. It's not about the bathroom scale. Forget about it. Forget about your weight or what other people think or say about your weight. Free your mind from all that, embracing instead the vision that you can be fit *and* free, even if you are not fat-free. I want you to get excited about the things you are going to do, the things you will learn about yourself, and the things that will help you live a long, happy life.

In each of the following chapters, we'll discuss crucial aspects of fitness and fatness, and provide an active step in a progressive program of learning and activity. It's an eight-week program, but if you need more time for one step, take it. Make it your program. Some parts of it will challenge you, taxing your emotions and your body, but these challenges are part of life. I like challenges myself because only by taking them on can I hope to be a winner. I want you to be a winner, too—a winner in the game of life.

CHAPTER 2

Week 1: The Motion Solution

Taking the First Crucial Steps in Your Personal Activity Program

In her wonderful poem "The Summer Day," poet Mary Oliver asks, "Tell me, what is it you plan to do with your one wild and precious life?" What a powerful and passionate question! It deserves an equally powerful and passionate answer. Have you taken charge of your own physical, metabolic, and emotional life? If not, why not start today, treating your one and only life with the great care it deserves? During this first week of your program, you'll learn how these three areas of your life fit together.

Start Living the Life You Have Always Wanted

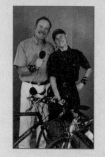 Trained as a psychotherapist, Dan Rudd had spent 30 years helping people achieve greater emotional health and studying the relationship between emotions and physical health. Then one day, in 1991, Dan confronted Mary Oliver's question head on.

In October of that year, Dan and his wife, Amy, went to Hawaii to cheer on a friend as she swam 2.4 miles in the ocean, rode her bike 112 miles through the lava fields, and then ran 26.2 miles in the race known as the Hawaii Ironman Triathlon. There was a magical quality to the day as Dan soaked up the excitement of the athletes and the spectators, and the natural beauty of the Kona Coast. Throughout the day, Dan could feel the tickle of desire that some day he might compete in this incredible event, but he could not overcome the fearful thought, "I am not as strong as these people. I could never find the time to train because my career and family demand all my time." On the plane ride home, Dan read a book I had given him: *The Road to Kona Never Ends*, by Patrick McCary, about people's aspirations to achieve their best-ever performance in the Hawaii Ironman Triathlon. That book inspired Dan to believe that some day he would compete in the Ironman.

Finally, desire began to win the battle with fear. Over the next nine years, Dan gradually set aside more time for exercise and started entering short races. When he confided his Ironman dream to me, I told him he needed to run a marathon. He agreed. Another friend offered to ride with him in a century ride, a 100-mile bike trip. Dan was lucky because his family fully supported his dream and accompanied him to events.

Dan's sons started out as volunteers at the races, handing out water to the athletes; then they began entering the races themselves. His wife, Amy, always stood at the finish line, greeting Dan with a hug and a smile. It didn't matter to his family that Dan finished far back in the pack; they celebrated his success just participating in the events. And in June 1999, Dan and his family traveled to Lake Placid, New York, where his dream came true as he completed the 2.4-mile swim, the 112-mile bike ride, and the 26.2-mile run at the Ironman USA Triathlon.

As a medical practitioner, Dan knew that fitness consists of metabolic, physical, and emotional elements. Obviously, he needed physical training and strength to complete the long Ironman race, but he also needed the emotional strength to overcome fear, doubt, weariness, and pain. You'll need emotional strength, too, as you start living the life you have always wanted.

Choosing a new direction for your "wild and precious life" and taking the first steps in that new direction are the most important decisions you'll ever make. It begins with commitment, believing in yourself, and "thinking" yourself into your new life before you actually do it.

Where's Your Starting Point?

Before you take your first step toward greater fitness, I want you this week to figure out your current levels of metabolic, physical, and emotional fitness. This means carrying out some self-assessments of where you are now. Only then can you set realistic goals for yourself. You're unique, your body is unique, and so will be the activity program you design. In this chapter, I give you some tools to start understanding aspects of your own personal health and fitness so that you will, at the end, have developed your own special vision of what changes you can make to enhance your life over the next eight weeks. Once you have completed the activities in this chapter, you will possess a clearer picture of your own unique biological makeup and will have taken the first, most crucial steps toward improved health and fitness.

Forget the Fat

Before you do anything else, I am going to ask you to do something that may surprise you. If you are like most people who carry extra fat, you quite probably worry or even stress about it. Well, I want you to stop thinking about fat right now. Stop reading about fat, stop calculating fat, and stop looking at fat in the mirror and defining yourself as a fat person. Because only you can choose the life you want to live, only you can stop living the life of a fat person and start living the life of somebody in touch with his or her metabolic, physical, and emotional fitness. Instead of thinking about fat, how fat you are, and how much fat you want to lose, and identifying yourself as a fat person, think instead about your health and fitness. Instead of doing things that remind you of how fat you are, stop and do things that help you think about how fit you can become. Believe me, you'll be doing yourself a big favor if you can eject that "fat" tape and replace it with a "fit" tape.

U.S. Government Subsidizes Weight Loss Industry

In the year 2002, the U.S. government established a new beachhead on its war on fatness when the Internal Revenue Service recognized obesity as a disease. "Weigh less and pay less? IRS adds new deductions," proclaimed headlines on the front page of most major daily newspapers. Now taxpayers would be allowed to deduct weight-loss expenses as a medical deduction, paving the way for insurance companies and government medical care programs to offer coverage for obesity treatments.

Why would the government award tax deductions for programs such as classic weight-loss programs with high failure rates? Typical weight-loss programs incur a 90 percent failure rate in the first year and a 99 percent failure rate over a 5 year period.[1] This development goes beyond the disproved notion that obesity causes disease, insisting that it itself is a disease. As a result, the U.S. government is subsidizing the weight-loss industry, one of the industries most responsible for the prevalence of obesity.

Fit *and* Fat

Activity 2.1: Play the Fit Tape, Not the Fat Tape

Working through the 8 weeks of the Fit *and* Fat program will teach you how to live in a way that puts you in touch with your metabolic, emotional, and physical health. But first you have to decide that you want to go in that direction. I know it's not easy because you've been bombarded all your life with "fat is bad" messages that have reinforced your image of yourself as a fat person, probably without you even realizing it. Thinking of yourself as a fat person will only perpetuate behaviors that do not contribute to your health—for example, dieting. Consider this list of behaviors that keep us living the life of a fat person and the better behaviors that can help you start living the life you have always wanted. Can you add to the lists? Can you discipline yourself to replace "fat behaviors" with "fit behaviors"?

Fat Behaviors	Fit Behaviors
Read a magazine article on fitness.	Read a magazine article on dieting.
Join a diet or weight-loss group in which you talk about diets and how to lose weight.	Join an athletic club where you meet people who talk about sports and exercise.
Add another diet book to your library.	Replace all those diet books with ones on your favorite activities.
Shop for clothes that hide the fat.	Shop for clothes that help you move.
Spend money on fat-loss solutions.	Rebudget your money for a fitness toy.
Prefer friends living the lives of fat people.	Hang out with friends who live the life you want.
Study your fat in the mirror.	Look at your muscles in the mirror.
Hire a diet/nutritional counselor/advisor.	Hire a personal trainer.
Deprive yourself of food.	Eat when you feel hungry.
Vacation at a health farm.	Plan an activity holiday.

Start a new blank book or note pad and call it your personal fitness log. This week you should start recording lots of facts about yourself in a notebook. On the first page, list your new "Fit Behaviors."

Where Did Our Preoccupation with Fat Come From?

Ironically, a century ago, people looked on fatness as a sign of health, wealth, and happiness. Those who carried a lot of fat would live longer and enjoy life more. Less likely to engage in back-breaking labor, they would fare better during leaner times and stand a better chance of surviving disease. For women, fatness would help them to survive childbirth and bear many children. In even more distant times, between 50,000 and 10,000 years B.C.E. when our ancestors lived a hunter-gatherer lifestyle, individuals who easily gained and stored fat outlived those who didn't. Researchers see the evolution of our genes at this time as the root of modern obesity: Ancient genetic selection programmed us to be as fat as our environment allows[2,3]. In ancient times, fat was good.

Today, however, we view fat as something bad, a condition that contributes chronic, or lifestyle, diseases as well as bad health and a shortened life span.

Only recently have we started caring about and measuring weight and fatness, beginning around the turn of the century when the life insurance companies launched what has now become a harmful obsession. Insurers wanted a means of classifying people that would enable them to identify those who were the most risky to insure. Without really knowing where to start, they measured obvious characteristics: height and weight. All our modern standards for defining and measuring fatness and acceptable weights trace their origins to data collected at this time.

We apply our modern fatness standards to every individual. But think about it. How can you possibly classify the entire population according to a single standard for relationship of weight to height? That's crazy. Think back to our two dogs, the Greyhound and the St. Bernard. Of course, a fat Greyhound would look odd, but so would a skinny St. Bernard. We readily accept individual differences in our pets. Why don't we do the same then for ourselves and stop imposing strict standards that don't take into account genetic heritage, biological makeup, race, level of athleticism, age, sex, and so on?

Those Crazy Height-Weight Tables

Height-weight tables and their recommendations concerning ideal weights do not provide you with any meaningful information about your health. As we learned in Chapter 1, maintaining a so-called "ideal weight" cannot ensure against disease and an early death. Only fitness can decrease your risks. So why do we rely on those old tables?

In his book *Big Fat Lies,* Glenn Gaesser sketches the history of the height and weight tables, first published between 1897 and 1912 by the life insurance industry. The tables showed the average weights of males and females in different age groups and identified those weighing more than 20 percent above the average for their age as being at risk of early death. Over the years, the criteria for what constitutes overweight have decreased.

Despite 30 years of research into weight and health, there is still no scientific evidence to prove a causal link between weight and health, and the scientific community remains divided on the role of weight in the development of disease. Nevertheless, the U.S. government published its own height-weight tables in 1980, 1985, 1990, and 1995, along with health guidelines that promote a narrow definition of the "ideal weight," classifying anyone above that narrow band as "overweight" or "obese." The classification relies on calculations of Body Mass Index (BMI), a mathematical formula that relates weight to height. Basically, the heavier you are for your height, the higher your BMI is. The higher the BMI is, the more overweight you are. A BMI of 25 or more indicates "overweight," and 30 or more indicates "obese." This applies to both men and women.

If you are interested in knowing whether you fall into one of these categories, use the following table to determine whether you are above the threshold weights for "overweight" and "obese" for your height. The metric and nonmetric math for calculating your exact BMI is given after the table. Here's an important point: BMI does not allow for variations in bone, fat, muscle, and organ weight. Therefore, a very athletic person with a high proportion of muscle might have a BMI in the "overweight" category, while a person with little muscle mass but a lot of fat could have an ideal BMI. In other words, BMI does not provide a reliable measure of fitness and health.

Threshold Weights for "Overweight" and "Obese" According to Height

| Height in Inches (cm) | Body Weight in Pounds (kg) | |
	BMI 25	BMI 30
58(147)	119(54)	143(65)
59(150)	124(56)	148(67)
60(152)	128(58)	153(70)
61(155)	132(60)	158(72)

Height in Inches (cm)	Body Weight in Pounds (kg)	
	BMI 25	BMI 30
62(157)	136(62)	164(74)
63(160)	141(64)	169(77)
64(163)	145(66)	174(79)
65(165)	150(68)	180(82)
66(168)	155(70)	186(84)
67(170)	159(72)	191(87)
68(173)	164(74)	197(89)
69(175)	169(77)	203(92)
70(178)	174(79)	207(94)
71(180)	179(81)	215(98)
72(183)	184(83)	221(100)
73(185)	189(86)	227(103)
74(188)	194(88)	233(106)
75(191)	200(91)	240(109)
76(193)	205(93)	246(111)

(National Institutes of Health, Clinical Guidelines)

Math for Calculation of Body Mass Index

Metric conversion formula = Weight (kg) ÷ Height (m)^2

Example: A person who a weight of 78.93 kg and is 177 cm tall has a BMI of 25:

Weight (78.93 kg) ÷ Height (1.77m)2 = 25

Nonmetric conversion formula = (Weight [pounds] ÷ Height [inches]^2) × 703

Example: A person who weighs 164 pounds and is 68 inches (or 5 feet, 8 inches) tall has a BMI of 25:

(Weight [164 pounds] ÷ Height [68 inches]^2) × 703 = 25

(National Institutes of Health, Clinical Guidelines)

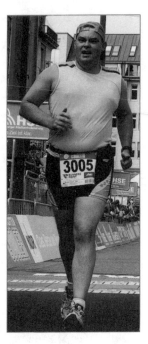

Kevin Brown, officially obese with a BMI of 33.3, crossing the finishing line of the Holsten City Man Olympic Distance Triathlon in Hamburg in 2002. A talented swimmer, Kevin took part in a team long distance triathlon at the world-famous Ironman course at Roth in Germany, swimming 3.8km in 1 hour and 8 minutes, placing him seventy-sixth out of an international field of 173 competitors.

Fat Trap: Did BMI Make You Overweight Overnight?

In June 1998, half the American population went to bed at a "healthy" weight, only to awaken the next morning to learn that, overnight, they became overweight or obese.

Before June 1998, the generally accepted BMI cut-off point for determining overweight was set at 27.8 for men and 27.3 for women, based on the National Health and Nutrition Survey (NHAMES II), a government-sponsored study carried out on 20,000 people between 1976 and 1980. These cut-off points were _arbitrarily_ set at the top 15 percent of individuals in a database of 20- to 29-year-old Americans. In other words, if you weighed the same as the heaviest 15 percent of 20- to 29-year-olds, you were automatically overweight or obese.[4]

In June 1998, the U.S. government issued the first Federal Obesity Clinical Guidelines. These reclassified overweight as anything over a BMI of 25, and obesity as anything over a BMI of 30. These new guidelines classify 55 percent of the American population (almost 100 million people) as overweight or obese.

Futile Fat Measurements

So if the BMI doesn't help us think about fat, what does? There are numerous ways of measuring body fatness, such as skin-fold thickness measurements, bioelectrical impedance (such as when using a set of home scales), infrared interactance, and even underwater weighing. If you visited a medical laboratory, you might even find densitometry, radiography, magnetic resonance imaging, dual-energy x-ray absorptiometry, photon absorptiometry, or total body electrical conductivity. Whatever the technique, you end up with percentages of muscle versus fat. One table sets these supposedly "ideal" fat percentages.

Suggested "Ideal" Ranges of Body Fat According to Age and Gender

Age	Males	Females
10 to 30	10 to 18 percent	20 to 25 percent
31 to 40	13 to 19 percent	21 to 27 percent
41 to 50	14 to 20 percent	22 to 28 percent
51 to 60	16 to 20 percent	22 to 30 percent
60+	17 to 21 percent	22 to 31 percent

However, percentages of fat mean about as much as the BMI. Neither your weight nor your height nor your body composition and proportion of fat to lean mass will tell you anything meaningful about your health. The idea of measuring fatness to assess fitness came, in large part, from exercise scientists who study body composition in athletes and who have assumed that athletes function well because of their generally low body fat percentages rather than because of their high amount of lean mass. The body fat standards may apply to athletes, but they don't mean much for a typical person. In fact, no scientifically valid guidelines exist for applying percentages of fat to the overall fit and healthy population.

Your health does not depend on how much fat you have, but on your metabolic, physical, and emotional fitness. Fat is just the padding on the outside and does not accurately reflect what's going on inside your body. All this talk about an "obesity epidemic" comes from scientists, insurance companies, the fashion industry, the weight-loss business, and, most recently, our own government, all of whom blame too much fat rather than too little fitness as the ultimate villain. They're all wrong. Fitness, not fatness, is the real issue.

It's Fitness, Not Fatness, That Really Counts: Lorraine's Story

When Lorraine realized that fitness, not fatness, is the real issue, amazing things happened in her life. Here's what she says:

I tried measuring fat, but it did not work. It was absolutely the wrong focus for my life. As soon as I moved away from this pointless exercise, things started to change. My whole life, I was told I was too fat, so I did everything I could to lose fat. Inevitably, I didn't lose any fat at all; I only gained it.

After I started focusing on fitness rather than fatness, things began to change. Yes, I lost about 20 pounds and dropped about 5 percent in body fat percentage, but I am still 38 percent fat and I have a high BMI. If I obsessed over this, I would just get depressed, but if I look at how my fitness has improved, I feel exhilarated.

Two years ago, when I started focusing on fitness rather than weight and fat, I could hardly run. At the beginning of my campaign to get fit, I ran for two minutes and then walked for five. That was all I could manage. I gradually built it up, and after 6 months I entered my first triathlon, where I ran for more than 30 minutes and totally shocked myself. This year, when I ran my first marathon, I ran for nearly five hours. To me it's quite clear what changed: When I just wanted to lose the fat, I failed. After I switched to thinking more about fitness and not worrying about the fat, I began to succeed totally and utterly beyond my wildest dreams.

Fixate on Your Fitness

What, exactly, do we mean by "fitness"? Like "beauty," it can mean different things to different people—in fact, the term spans a broad range of levels and types of fitness. It is not a static point or an on-off button. It is a continuum between zero-level of fitness to your personal, individual best-ever level of fitness. Think of it, then, as a sort of sliding scale from 0 to 10. Your 10 will differ from mine; Dan Rudd's will differ from Lorraine's.

Don't compare yourself to me or to anyone else. Your own fitness is unique to you and your specific biological makeup. Fitness is also activity-specific. Venus Williams is perfectly fit for tennis, but she would not fare well if asked to race against the world's fittest bicyclist, Lance Armstrong. I doubt whether Lance could return Venus's serve, either, although it would be fun to watch him try. Fitness is also fuel-specific. You can be fit at metabolizing carbohydrates but not fit at oxidizing fats, or you can be fit at using oxygen but not at resynthesizing lactate. Finally, fitness is function-specific. You can be fit at lifting heavy weights doing bench presses at your health club, but you can struggle to lift a bag of groceries up to a high shelf.

Are you fit? You would probably answer, "Sort of" or "It depends." It depends on where you are on your own fitness continuum, plus where you are with respect to specific activities, fuels, and functions. As you work out and participate more in physical activities that you love, you move toward 10, while if you slack off and do less, you fall back toward 0. Your answer also might take a certain activity into account. You might feel fit for a 5km (3.1 mile) run but not at all fit for a 26-mile (42.02km) marathon.

For our purposes, we will focus on three different kinds of fitness—the fitness triad.

The Total Body Fitness Triad

Any fitness program should address all three components: metabolic, physical, and emotional fitness. Otherwise, you're not taking into account all the features that contribute to a long, happy, healthful life.

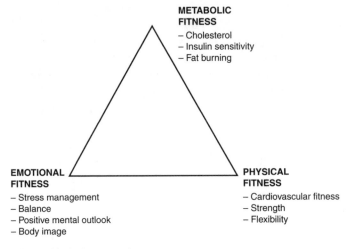

The total body fitness triad.

- **Metabolic fitness.** The processes that digest, utilize, and store energy; release energy from storage; and control appetite and satiety signals are all working well. Healthy levels of glucose tolerance, insulin sensitivity, blood fats, and fat metabolism.

- **Physical fitness.**
  Health:
  - Cardiorespiratory endurance
  - Muscular strength
  - Muscular endurance
  - Balance and coordination
  - Flexibility

  Skills:
  - Coordination
  - Balance
  - Power
  - Speed
  - Agility
  - Reaction time
- **Emotional fitness.** Ability to cope with stress, build positive relationships, deal with change, maintain balance in life.

Do you see the word *fat* in the triad? No, because fitness does not depend on lack of fatness. Many fitness and medical experts measure body fat as a way of defining fitness. Some even use it as the sole criterion for fitness. In fact, society has placed so much emphasis on the measurement of body fat (skinfold calipers, underwater weighing, bioelectrical impedance, infrared methods, and so on) that most people automatically accept them as tests of fitness. It all springs from the same prejudice that body fat is bad and that lean tissue (muscles, bones, and so on) is good. As we've learned, fat in and of itself is not bad. It is an essential part of good health. And as the evidence in Chapter 1 showed, high percentages of body fat do *not* cause decreased longevity or poor health. You can be fat and have perfectly good health, provided that you include all components of the triad.

No fitness program should focus on the goal of losing body weight and body fat. Instead, you should concentrate on the goal of gaining metabolic, physical, and emotional fitness, and the health improvements that occur as a result. Never make the mistake of measuring fitness and health improvements in terms of weight loss or fat reduction. Neither science nor common sense links either body weight or body composition to fitness.

Metabolic Fitness

Forget the numbers on your bathroom scale and pay attention instead to the numbers that mean something: your cholesterol, your blood pressure, and your insulin sensitivity. Those numbers reflect metabolic fitness (more about how to obtain these numbers in Chapter 5). You can also learn much about your metabolism through observation, which you will begin later in this chapter with an activity. You'll use some of these observations in Chapters 4 and 5 to help you piece together an understanding of your own unique metabolism.

Metabolism includes all of your body's energy activities, the chemical reactions and processes that occur every second of your life to provide energy for vital processes and movement. According to Professor Glenn A. Gaesser, Ph.D., of the University of Virginia, "Being metabolically fit means having a metabolism that maximizes vitality and minimizes the risk of disease—particularly those diseases that are influenced by lifestyle, such as heart disease, type II diabetes, and cancer."[5] Recent studies indicate that you might even add Alzheimer's to that list. Measures of metabolic fitness reveal how well or how efficiently your metabolism works. We'll talk more about metabolic fitness and its importance later. For now, though, just note that it is a relatively new part of the fitness puzzle, one that you can measure in a lot of ways, including insulin sensitivity and blood sugar levels, resting metabolic rates, blood pressure, and cholesterol levels. Metabolic fitness is such an important part of fitness that I'll talk about it in detail, including ways you can measure it, in Chapter 5.

Activity 2.2: Monitor Your Metabolism

Unless you find out about your own unique metabolism, you'll never achieve the goal of improving it. This week I want you to observe how well your metabolism functions right now. During the next seven days, monitor your metabolism by asking yourself these questions and noting your observations in your personal fitness log.

1. Do I eat less than other family members/friends but tend to gain weight more easily?
2. How does my appetite compare to that of family members/friends?
3. Do I tend to eat more quickly or more slowly than others?
4. Do I eat standing up or on the go?
5. In terms of body temperature, am I a cold person or a warm person?
6. Do I experience poor circulation and cold hands/feet when I'm not moving?
7. How long do I go between meals without feeling hungry?

Activity 2.2. *continued*

8. Does hunger make me irritable?

9. What times of day do I get hungry, and when do I feel the hungriest?

10. Does my body warm up after eating a meal?

11. What kind of foods do I crave the most and when?

12. Have I ever put on a lot of weight or lost a lot of weight? Why?

13. When do I feel the most energized?

14. Do some kinds of foods make me feel energized, while others make me feel sluggish?

15. Do I find it harder to lose weight these days compared to some years ago, even though I eat less?

16. Are there any foods that disagree with my system and result in abdominal bloating, gas, or diarrhea?

17. Do I have energy for the things I want to do?

For now, just keep a note of anything you notice about your metabolism. You will use this information in Chapters 4 and 5 when I deal specifically with your energy balancing processes and metabolism.

Physical Fitness

Fitness training includes two major components: health improvement and skill improvement. Physical health improvements include getting stronger, building endurance, and increasing flexibility and mobility. Your body weight and composition will most likely change when you do this type of training. Physical skill improvements include developing more powerful muscles that respond more quickly and provide you with greater coordination and balance and agility. Improvements in your physical fitness through training will reward you with a longer, more vital, and higher-quality life.

Because moderate-intensity exercise is safe for most people, you can start increasing your level of physical activity right away. If you know you have a medical problem such as heart disease or diabetes, you should check with your doctor first. If not, you can fill out the Physical Activity Readiness Questionnaire (PAR-Q) that follows. Your answers will help you decide whether you need to see a doctor or can safely begin an exercise program.

Activity 2.3: Do I Need to See My Doctor? Take the PAR-Q Test

Carefully read the following Physical Activity Readiness Questionnaire (PAR-Q) and answer each question honestly. If you answer Yes to one or more questions, talk with your doctor before you increase your physical activity; take the questionnaire along to the consultation.

Physical Activity Readiness
Questionnaire - PAR-Q
(revised 2002)

PAR-Q & YOU

(A Questionnaire for People Aged 15 to 69)

Regular physical activity is fun and healthy, and increasingly more people are starting to become more active every day. Being more active is very safe for most people. However, some people should check with their doctor before they start becoming much more physically active.

If you are planning to become much more physically active than you are now, start by answering the seven questions in the box below. If you are between the ages of 15 and 69, the PAR-Q will tell you if you should check with your doctor before you start. If you are over 69 years of age, and you are not used to being very active, check with your doctor.

Common sense is your best guide when you answer these questions. Please read the questions carefully and answer each one honestly: check YES or NO.

YES	NO		
☐	☐	1.	Has your doctor ever said that you have a heart condition <u>and</u> that you should only do physical activity recommended by a doctor?
☐	☐	2.	Do you feel pain in your chest when you do physical activity?
☐	☐	3.	In the past month, have you had chest pain when you were not doing physical activity?
☐	☐	4.	Do you lose your balance because of dizziness or do you ever lose consciousness?
☐	☐	5.	Do you have a bone or joint problem (for example, back, knee or hip) that could be made worse by a change in your physical activity?
☐	☐	6.	Is your doctor currently prescribing drugs (for example, water pills) for your blood pressure or heart condition?
☐	☐	7.	Do you know of <u>any other reason</u> why you should not do physical activity?

If

you

answered

YES to one or more questions

Talk with your doctor by phone or in person BEFORE you start becoming much more physically active or BEFORE you have a fitness appraisal. Tell your doctor about the PAR-Q and which questions you answered YES.

- You may be able to do any activity you want — as long as you start slowly and build up gradually. Or, you may need to restrict your activities to those which are safe for you. Talk with your doctor about the kinds of activities you wish to participate in and follow his/her advice.
- Find out which community programs are safe and helpful for you.

NO to all questions

If you answered NO honestly to <u>all</u> PAR-Q questions, you can be reasonably sure that you can:
- start becoming much more physically active – begin slowly and build up gradually. This is the safest and easiest way to go.
- take part in a fitness appraisal – this is an excellent way to determine your basic fitness so that you can plan the best way for you to live actively. It is also highly recommended that you have your blood pressure evaluated. If your reading is over 144/94, talk with your doctor before you start becoming much more physically active.

DELAY BECOMING MUCH MORE ACTIVE:
- if you are not feeling well because of a temporary illness such as a cold or a fever – wait until you feel better; or
- if you are or may be pregnant – talk to your doctor before you start becoming more active.

PLEASE NOTE: If your health changes so that you then answer YES to any of the above questions, tell your fitness or health professional. Ask whether you should change your physical activity plan.

<u>Informed Use of the PAR-Q</u>: The Canadian Society for Exercise Physiology, Health Canada, and their agents assume no liability for persons who undertake physical activity, and if in doubt after completing this questionnaire, consult your doctor prior to physical activity.

No changes permitted. You are encouraged to photocopy the PAR-Q but only if you use the entire form.

NOTE: If the PAR-Q is being given to a person before he or she participates in a physical activity program or a fitness appraisal, this section may be used for legal or administrative purposes.

"I have read, understood and completed this questionnaire. Any questions I had were answered to my full satisfaction."

NAME _____

SIGNATURE _____ DATE _____

SIGNATURE OF PARENT _____ WITNESS _____
or GUARDIAN (for participants under the age of majority)

Note: This physical activity clearance is valid for a maximum of 12 months from the date it is completed and becomes invalid if your condition changes so that you would answer YES to any of the seven questions.

CSEP
SCPE © Canadian Society for Exercise Physiology   Supported by: ▌◆▌ Health   Santé
                                                                  Canada   Canada

Your Heart Rate

The most important muscle in your body is your heart muscle. Although you can't see or feel it, you can find out a lot about it. You can take your pulse manually, of course, but I strongly recommend that you do what I do: Use an inexpensive heart rate monitor that will display and even record your heart rate before, during, and after activities.

Your heart rate and your pulse rate are usually, but not necessarily, equal. "Heart rate" refers to the electrical impulses that cause your heart to beat, but "pulse rate" refers only to the movement of blood through your arteries. Heart rate monitors use electrical changes of the heart as the signal, while manual pulse rate uses biomechanical blood flow of the heart as the signal. When you take your pulse manually, you're taking your "pulse rate."

Each time the left ventricle of the heart contracts, it pumps a surge of blood into the aorta and into the peripheral vessels of the arterial system. You can feel this stretch and subsequent recoil of the arterial wall during a complete cardiac cycle by applying light pressure with your fingers over any artery near the surface of the skin.

To measure your pulse manually, place two fingers over the inside surface of your wrist and lightly apply pressure. Wait quietly, moving your fingers until you feel the blood flow. You can also use arteries in the groin and the neck, but taking your pulse rate from your neck's carotid artery can slow your heart rate and sometimes give you a false reading.

Pulse can best be measured manually when you remain stationary, which makes this method less useful for those who are exercising. When you stop exercising to count your pulse, it almost immediately begins to drop (for some really fit people, it plummets like a stone). This leads to calculating an inaccurate pulse rate. It's common for the very fit to see their pulse drop a beat per second. That can result in a 10- to 15-beat error when counting manually.

The easiest way to get a manual result is to count the number of pulse waves during six seconds, adding a zero to that number to obtain beats per minute (bpm). For example, if in 6 seconds you count 8 beats, adding a 0 results in 80 beats per minute. Others prefer to count pulse for 10 seconds, multiplying that number by 6, or for 15 seconds, multiplying by 4. Accuracy of measurement is so important that I urge you to invest in a heart rate monitor. You'll never regret that investment.

Whether you do it manually or electronically, you want to make it a routine habit to measure your heart rate in beats per minute (bpm).

Your heart rate reflects how your body reacts to activity. For example, when I walk on flat terrain, my heart rate averages about 100 bpm. When I run fast, it increases to about 150 bpm. Clearly, hard running is more strenuous, causing my heart muscle to respond by increasing the flow of blood to the working muscles in my legs. On the other hand, while sitting here writing this book, I measure a heart rate of 60 bpm. My heart doesn't need to pump so much blood for this activity.

Activity 2.4: Measure Your Heart Rate

Now you're ready to take important heart rate measurements. Use the manual "pulse rate" method if you don't have a heart rate monitor. Record the result using the Heart Rate Log in Appendix F.

- **Resting heart rate.** This is your heart rate while sitting or at rest. This is an important indicator of your health and fitness. The lower this number is, the better. The normal range is 60 to 70, while a trained athlete might have a resting heart rate of as low as 50 bpm.

  1. Sit down.

  2. Relax for at least five minutes.

  3. Quiet yourself.

  4. Now count the number of heart beats per minute. This number is your resting heart rate, one of the best and easiest tests for assessing your current level of health. The lower the number is, the better your cardiac health is. My resting heart rate right now is 60 bpm.

  5. Record your own number in the Fit *and* Fat Heart Rate Log provided in Appendix F.

- **Delta heart rate.** This tells you the difference in your rate between lying down and standing up. The delta heart rate is an indicator of your heart health. The smaller the difference is between how hard your heart has to work between lying down and standing up, the better. A healthy delta heart rate is below 15 bpm.

  1. Lie down on your back for two minutes, relaxing and remaining still.

  2. At the end of two minutes, count and record your heart rate while lying down (L).

Activity 2.4. *continued*

3. Stand up in place and remain standing for two minutes.

4. At the end of this two-minute period, count your heart rate. This is your rate while standing (S).

5. Next, subtract your standing heart rate (S) from your lying down heart rate (L). The difference between these two numbers is your delta heart rate. For example, my standing heart rate is 78 bpm and my lying down heart rate is 65 bpm, with a differential of 13. The lower the DHR is, the better.

6. Record this information in the Fit *and* Fat Pulse Rate Log.

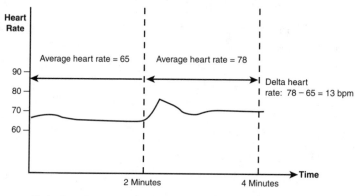

Delta heart rate.

- **Recovery heart rate.** The fitter you are, the faster your pulse rate recovers from a high rate. You can measure recovery heart rate several different ways, but the following works quite well:

   1. Select an enjoyable activity, such as walking, cycling, swimming, or any other relatively strenuous workout. Warm up to an effort level that you would describe as "moderate" (that is, you can maintain that level of intensity for several minutes with little to no pain).

   2. After performing this activity for five minutes at a steady level of effort, record your heart rate. This number is your steady state heart rate.

   3. At the end of a minimum of 5 minutes, stop the activity and stand in place calmly, waiting 60 seconds before counting your heart rate. This pulse rate number is your one-minute recovery pulse heart rate.

4. Next, stand in place for another 60 seconds and then count your heart rate again. This is your two-minute recovery heart rate.

5. Use the following Recovery Heart Rate table to help you calculate your recovery heart rate, and record your results in the Fit *and* Fat Heart Rate Log.

Your recovery heart rate for today is the difference between the steady state moderate-intensity pulse rate you maintained for the exercise period and your heart rate at the end of one minute and again at the end of two minutes. For example, my heart rate was 140 bpm when I was bicycling this morning. When we stopped at the end, I stood still for one minute while monitoring my pulse rate: At the end of 1 minute, it was 110 bpm. After I stood still for another minute, it dropped to 86 bpm. My 1-minute recovery was 30 bpm (140 − 110), and my 2-minute recovery was 54 bpm (140 − 86). As a guideline, your recovery heart rate should be more than 15 bpm. It's not uncommon to measure recovery rates of 60 to 70 bpm. The higher your recovery heart rate is, the better.

Recovery Heart Rate

Steady State Heart Rate Number	(−) Heart Rate After 60 Seconds	(=) Recovery Pulse Rate Number
One-minute recovery heart rate number:		
_____ bpm	− _____ bpm	= recovery heart rate
Two-minute recovery heart rate number:		
_____ bpm	− _____ bpm	= recovery heart rate

Find Out What Your Body Can Do

Now that you've looked at your heart and done a few tests, it's time to see what your body can do. The following will help you make a simple assessment of your physical fitness. You should do these tests now so that you can take them again at the end of the program and see how fit you've become. The first is the American Heart Association Everyday Fitness Test, designed to help you determine how fit you are for your everyday life. Complete the questionnaire and write the results in your personal fitness log.

Activity 2.5: American Heart Association Everyday Fitness Test

Aerobic Activities:

1. After walking up a flight of stairs, I feel:

   No discomfort   Short of breath

      1   2   3   4   5

2. After walking from gate to gate at the airport, I feel:

   No discomfort   Short of breath

      1   2   3   4   5

3. After walking from one end of the mall to the other, I feel:

   No discomfort   Short of breath

      1   2   3   4   5

Total points: _____

Strength Activities:

4. After lifting or carrying groceries, luggage, or other heavy items, I feel:

   No discomfort   Weak

      1   2   3   4   5

5. After pushing the vacuum cleaner or lawn mower, I feel:

   No discomfort   Weak

      1   2   3   4   5

6. After holding a small child for several minutes, I feel:

   No discomfort   Weak

      1   2   3   4   5

Total Points: _____

Mobility Activities:

7. When bending to tie my shoes, I feel:

   No discomfort   Weak

      1   2   3   4   5

8. When bending and stretching to make a bed, I feel:

No discomfort				Weak
1	2	3	4	5

9. When reaching for the top cabinet shelf, I feel:

No discomfort				Weak
1	2	3	4	5

Total Points: _____

What's the Score?

If your total score for any of the three fitness components was between 3 and 8, you're off to a good start. If you scored between 9 and 15, you're in the right place. The fitness tips you will be receiving over the next few months will help you boost your fitness level. Then you can do these exercises (and more strenuous ones!) with ease and comfort. Be sure to check with your doctor before beginning an exercise program.

Reprinted with permission from the American Heart Association Fitting in Fitness, copyright © 1997 by the American Heart Association. Published by Random House, Inc. Available from booksellers everywhere.

The next activity is a walking test developed at the Exercise Physiology and Nutrition Laboratory of the University of Massachusetts Medical Center. It's designed to be a measure of your cardiovascular (or heart) fitness. When you have completed the test, you compare your heart rate at the end of the test, and the time you took to complete the test, to data tables showing the relative performance for people your sex and age. You can find more information about the test at www.rockport.com.

Activity 2.6: Rockport One-Mile Fitness Walking Test

This test involves a one-mile walk during which you measure your heart rate and the time it takes to go that distance. You can compare your results to standard tables of time and heart rate for a person your age. You will find these in Appendix F.

1. Find a suitable place where you can walk a full measured mile on flat ground, preferably surfaced. Don't eat a heavy meal for at least three hours before the test (a snack is all right), and don't drink caffeinated drinks beforehand because caffeine can affect your heart rate.

Activity 2.6. *continued*

2. Dress in comfortable clothes and shoes. You will also need a watch to time yourself, and a pencil and a piece of paper to record your results.

3. Before you start, take your pulse, either manually or with a heart rate monitor; write it down.

4. Warm up for 5 to 10 minutes by walking until you feel loosened up and ready to go.

5. As soon as you are ready to go, note the time, or start your stopwatch, if you are using one. Then walk the mile at a brisk pace without stopping. Walk with a purpose as if you were heading for an appointment, but not so fast that you can't carry on a conversation.

6. At the end of the mile, note your time and take your pulse. Then walk at an easy pace for 5 to 10 minutes to cool down.

7. When you get home, compare your results to the data tables in Appendix F for your sex and age, and plot your one-mile time against your finishing heart rate to determine your relative fitness level.

Emotional Fitness

The most important muscle in our bodies, the heart muscle, diligently pumps nutrients and oxygen to every cell in the body 24 hours a day, 365 days a year for our entire lifetime. At the same time, the emotional "heart" pumps the nutrients of our feelings, inspiration, and motivation to every corner of our being.

In the Fit *and* Fat program, taking care of the emotional heart matters as much as caring for the physical heart. Learning about the "emotional zones" and how you can train your emotional heart will help you keep stress and emotional upset from harming your physical heart. By focusing on emotional fitness along with physical and metabolic fitness, you gain the power to achieve your goal of improving your health and improving your well-being. Remember, the Fit *and* Fat program is *not* a diet. It is *not* a temporary plan for achieving short-term goals. It *is* a new lifestyle for you that unites your biological makeup and your dreams for a life of better health and happiness.

Activity 2.7: Evaluate Your Emotions

Observe your emotional life for a week, pinpointing which parts of your life ignite good emotions and which parts spark bad emotions. Write any observations you make in your personal fitness log.

Good Emotions: When and Why

Relaxed: _____

Playful: _____

Carefree: _____

Generous: _____

Loved: _____

Happy: _____

Delighted: _____

Confident: _____

Powerful: _____

Enthusiastic: _____

Determined: _____

Impulsive: _____

Elated: _____

Fulfilled: _____

Grateful: _____

Helpful: _____

Needed: _____

Extravagant: _____

Impulsive: _____

Pleased: _____

Fabulous: _____

Contented: _____

Adventurous: _____

Secure: _____

Bad Emotions: When and Why

Angry: _____

Fearful: _____

Anxious: _____

Impatient: _____

Pessimistic: _____

Vulnerable: _____

Suspicious: _____

Cautious: _____

Gloomy: _____

Uncooperative: _____

Insecure: _____

Miserable: _____

Lost: _____

Resentful: _____

Helpless: _____

Depressed: _____

Apprehensive: _____

Exasperated: _____

Bored: _____

Envious: _____

Ugly: _____

Furious: _____

Irritated: _____

Problematic: _____

Stress creates real physical problems, not just mental ones. That's because what happens in our emotional heart greatly affects our physical heart and our whole body. For example, psychologists have long known that an accumulation of stressful life events can lead to poor health.

Stress can play a powerful role in your life. Often when we think of personal stressors—that is, things that stress us—we think of major events or even catastrophes. But even little daily things can bring about stress when added together.

Activity 2.8: Rating the Stressors in Your Life

Use the following test to determine the load of stressors in your life. Consider each of the following events. In Column A, indicate the number of times you have experienced each one during the last 12 months. Write your results in your personal fitness log.

Column A Number of Times Life-Changing Event	Column B Points	Column C (A × B)
___ 1. Entered college	50	___
___ 2. Married	77	___
___ 3. Had trouble with your boss	38	___
___ 4. Held a job while attending school	43	___
___ 5. Experienced the death of a spouse	87	___
___ 6. Experienced a major change in sleeping habits	34	___
___ 7. Experienced the death of a close family member	77	___
___ 8. Experienced a major change in eating habits	30	___
___ 9. Changed major field of study	41	___
___ 10. Revised personal habits	45	___
___ 11. Experienced the death of a close friend	68	___
___ 12. Found guilty of minor violations of the law	22	___
___ 13. Recognized an outstanding personal achievement	40	___
___ 14. Experienced pregnancy or fathered a pregnancy	68	___
___ 15. Experienced a major change in the health or behavior of family member	56	___

Column A Number of Times Life-Changing Event	Column B Points	Column C (A × B)
___ 16. Had sexual difficulties	58	___
___ 17. Had trouble with in-laws	42	___
___ 18. Experienced a major change in the number of family get-togethers	26	___
___ 19. Experienced a major change in financial state	53	___
___ 20. Gained a new family member	50	___
___ 21. Changed a residence or living conditions	42	___
___ 22. Experienced a major conflict or change in values	50	___
___ 23. Experienced a major change in church activities	36	___
___ 24. Reconciled with your mate	58	___
___ 25. Got fired from work	62	___
___ 26. Got divorced	76	___
___ 27. Changed to a different line of work	50	___
___ 28. Experienced a major change in the number of arguments with your spouse	50	___
___ 29. Experienced a major change in responsibilities at work	47	___
___ 30. Had your spouse begin or cease working outside the home	41	___
___ 31. Experienced a major change in working hours or conditions	42	___
___ 32. Separated from your mate	74	___
___ 33. Experienced a major change in the type or amount of recreation	37	___
___ 34. Experienced a major change in the use of drugs	52	___
___ 35. Took out a mortgage or loan of less than $10,000	52	___
___ 36. Experienced a major personal injury or illness	65	___
___ 37. Experienced a major change in the use of alcohol	46	___

Activity 2.8. *continued*

Column A Number of Times Life-Changing Event	Column B Points	Column C (A × B)
___ 38. Experienced a major change in social activities	43	____
___ 39. Experienced a major change in the amount of participation in school activities	38	____
___ 40. Experienced a major change in your amount of independence and responsibility	49	____
___ 41. Took a trip or a vacation	33	____
___ 42. Got engaged to be married	54	____
___ 43. Changed to a new school	50	____
___ 44. Changed dating habits	41	____
___ 45. Had trouble with school administration	44	____
___ 46. Broke off a marital engagement or steady relationship	60	____
___ 47. Experienced a major change in self-concept or self-awareness	57	____

To find your score on this scale, multiply the number in Column B by the number in Column A, and place it in Column C. Then total Column C. If your score totals 1,450 or higher, you are in the high category for developing an illness. If your total is 350 or less, you fall into the low category. The medium score is 900.

How well do you handle the stressful events that come along in your life? It's impossible to live in our modern world without experiencing the everyday stresses of commuting, balancing work and home life, managing the finances, and keeping up with the pace of life. Do you sometimes let things get to you, or do you glide through life unfazed? Here's a little quiz to help you think about how well you handle the stressful situations that come your way.

Activity 2.9: How Susceptible Are You to Stress?

Having looked at the stressors in your life, you can now consider how you manage stress in your life and how susceptible you may be to the negative effects of too much stress.

Stress Test (True or False)

___ 1. The cable repair company promised to arrive between 1 and 3, and here it is almost 4. You've called twice, only to get a recorded message. You can feel your anger rising and your heart beating faster.

___ 2. You have expensive tickets to a big game, and you're already running a little late. Your spouse is lingering over what to wear, though you've insisted twice that it's time to go. Suddenly you lose your patience and get angry.

___ 3. Things are a little shaky at work, and now you've been asked to come in for a meeting with your supervisor on Friday. You know you shouldn't let it get to you. Still, you can't help but be anxious. For the next two nights, you find yourself waking up with a feeling of dread.

___ 4. You've waited almost a half-hour for a table at a restaurant, and suddenly the host seems to be seating a party that arrived after yours. You feel your face burn and your muscles tense up with anger.

___ 5. In the middle of a phone conversation, a friend gets another call on call waiting and puts you on hold. Thirty seconds pass. With your anger mounting, you slam down the phone.

___ 6. It's been a long, hectic day, and you know you should take some time to relax and unwind, but you can't seem to slow down. Driving home, another driver almost cuts you off by mistake. You blast the horn and hold it down long enough to show how angry you are.

In each hypothetical situation, there are different ways to respond when something goes wrong. You can get mad when a driver inadvertently cuts you off, for instance, or you can shrug it off and remind yourself that you've done the same thing sometimes. You can slam down the phone, or you can wait until your friend gets back on the line and then gently say you'd rather have her call you back than put you on hold.

Activity 2.9. *continued*

Look back over your answers. If you answered True to most questions, chances are you're what psychologists call a hot reactor. Instead of staying cool when problems arise, your heart rate accelerates, your muscles tense up, and you feel your anger surging. The more times you answered True, the more important it is to find healthy ways to defuse stress.

(Source: Active Living Every Day: 20 Weeks to Lifelong Vitality, *by Steven N. Blair, editor; Andrea L. Dunn, Ph.D.; Bess H. Marcus, Ph.D.; Kenneth H. Cooper; and Peter Jaret, published by Human Kinetics (T), April 2001)*

Week 1 Summary

During this first week, I introduced you to the start of your Fit *and* Fat personal activity program. The first steps are the most important ones. Having taken some basic tests, you should have a fairly good idea of your current level of fitness—not only your physical fitness, but your metabolic and your emotional fitness as well. You've tried out some activities based on heart rate, and you've really begun to understand your own individual physiology. You've taken the time to examine the life you lead at the moment and the one you want to lead in the future.

You are well on the way to major life changes. Remember, though, that you want to change things one step at a time. It's better to change one thing and do that well 100 times than to change 100 things and do them all poorly. Next week, you'll learn more about how your body works. We'll introduce you to the language of the heart and a system of working out based around your own heart. I hope you keep up the small changes you've made this week. They are really important. But above all, I hope you are having fun!

CHAPTER 3

Week 2: The Language of the Heart

Monitoring Your Heart Rate for Maximum Results

Maybe you're wondering by now why the Fit *and* Fat program is a Heart Zones Program and why you've been asked to make some measurements of your heart rate. Well, the heart is the most important muscle in the body and during this week, you will learn a surprising amount about your fitness and your fatness through the use of a simple and inexpensive heart rate monitor. Here's what Mike Senning learned about his fitness and fatness.

Listening to Your Heart: Mike's Story

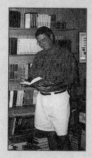 Mike Senning worked hard for 35 years in the publishing industry, earning an early retirement that would allow him to spend his time doing what he loved most: spending time with his family, golfing, fishing, and sailing. At age 58, he left his company with a monthly pension he planned to supplement by consulting to authors two days per week, leaving the rest of the time for all those activities he'd neglected throughout his career. Mike soon got into a routine of a one-hour early morning walk with the family dog and his wife, followed by a few hours of work and then a round of golf or a couple hours at the health club. One or two days a week, he biked down to the beach near his home in Wellfleet, Massachusetts, to fish for bass and bluefish; on weekends and holidays, he often crewed on a friend's yacht. Finally, he was living the life he had always wanted.

Just one thing kept nagging Mike: With all this activity, why wasn't he losing those extra pounds he'd gained over the years? After all, he was getting plenty of exercise and he was watching what he ate. The American College of Sports Medicine recommends 30 minutes of moderate physical activity per day, and he was getting a lot more than that, with taking his daily walks, golfing, using the rowing machine at the health club, biking to the beach, and sailing. Thinking a diet might do the trick, he tried the Zone Diet and then the Atkins Diet. But neither worked in the long run. Mike was hungry all the time, was grumpy, had no energy for his daily activities, and just couldn't stop thinking about food all the time. It was ridiculous. This wasn't the life he wanted to lead. Every 5 to 10 pounds he lost would creep back on when he went back to his normal day-to-day life.

One day at the athletic club, Mike shared his frustration with his friend Alan. Alan, an extremely fit 65-year-old, said something that surprised Mike: "You're doing a lot of things, but you're not actually doing the *right* things, exercise that challenges and pushes your body. All your activities are pretty low-key." Mike shook his head. "What do you mean? I get more exercise than most people. I'm always on the move. What do you mean by the *right* exercise?" That's when Alan showed Mike his heart rate monitor, saying, "I know that my workout is the right intensity for me because I can see exactly what my heart is doing. I regularly get up to 142 beats per minute on the treadmill. I bet you don't get yours past 120 with any of the activities you do, especially golfing."

Alan persuaded Mike to try the heart rate monitor for a week. What did he have to lose? As it turned out, he lost a lot. He lost all his illusions about exercise. His heart rate was 100 during his morning walk, 112 to 115 when he was rowing or mowing the lawn, and around 90 during a round of golf (110 when putting). Sailing was quite relaxing, apart from short bursts of activity that would get his heart rate up to 115 for 2 to 3 minutes. These numbers taught Mike that, despite all his activity, he wasn't getting any quality training time. He was not raising his heart rate enough to stimulate his body to get fitter.

Mike decided to buy an inexpensive heart rate monitor and try a little experiment. What would happen to his levels of fitness and fatness if he added just a little more strenuous fitness training to his schedule? As a first step, he spent 20 minutes working out on the rowing machine and then the elliptical trainer. Mike found it so hard to get his heart rate up to his aerobic zone around 140 that he managed just 5 minutes at that level on each piece of equipment. Gradually, over the weeks, he built himself up to 140 for 15 minutes on each. After one month, the results amazed him. He could see and feel significant changes in his body shape. His back and stomach were much firmer, and the spare tire around his midsection had deflated. He felt more energetic than he had felt for years. Carrying boxes of equipment to the boat did not faze him, and he even tightened his belt a notch. Mike wasn't spending any more time exercising, but thanks to the heart rate monitor, he had learned the language of his heart and was treating it better than he ever had.

Learning the Language of the Heart

This week I want you to learn the language of the heart, the one muscle on which your physical, metabolic, and emotional well-being depends. Training without listening to your heart is like trying to drive a high-performance car without a tachometer, the gauge that measures revolutions per minute (rpm). Without a tachometer, you don't know how hard your engine is working and when to shift to another gear to avoid damaging your engine. If you don't know how hard your heart is working, you don't know whether your physical activity program will give you the benefits you want.

Last week you took some simple measurements of your heart rate. Now you need to understand a bit more about how the heart works and why it is vital for you to base your individualized Fit *and* Fat training program on your own heart's parameters. You will learn what to look for when you shop for a heart rate monitor. Then you will learn how to determine the upper limit of your own heart rate range and how to set up personalized training zones. Finally, you will go out and train using your heart rate as your guide.

The power of the heart drives every joyful life. Because this great cardiac muscle remains in constant dialogue with every cell in your body and every corner of your mind, you should want to master its language. As with any new language, learning the language of the heart requires listening, interpretation, comprehension, understanding, and response. If you were to take up Japanese and become a "student" of the language, you would take classes that would progress from single words to phrases, sentences, and eventually paragraphs and stories. The same sort of progression applies to the language of the heart. The individual heartbeat is a word, and 75 years of heartbeats create the story of a life.

The Miracle of the Heart Rate Monitor

Two thousand years ago, Chinese doctors listened to the language of the heart by feeling the pulse. Two hundred years ago, European physicians began hearing it through stethoscopes. Today anyone can monitor the language of the heart with an amazing and inexpensive device called a heart rate monitor. This valuable tool works something like a radio. A strap that goes around your chest and rests snugly under the breast line contains electrodes that detect and transmit the tiny electric pulse of your heartbeat. A wristwatch-like receiver picks up and displays your heart rate at that moment. When you're sitting in a chair reading a book, it will display perhaps 50 to 85 bpm. When you spring to catch a bus, it will escalate to a higher number, perhaps 100 to 120 bpm. A personal heart rate monitor is the most accurate way to monitor your heart's activity outside a laboratory. A good one costs no more than a good pair of athletic shoes and is normally available in any sports shop where you would shop for good athletic shoes. In terms of your fitness and health, it could be the best investment you ever make.

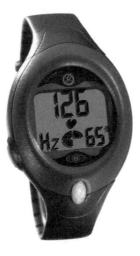

A heart rate monitor. When at rest, the lower your heart rate number the better. When exercising, your heart rate gives you an exertion rating, or an indication of how hard your body is working.

Why Use a Heart Rate Monitor?

A heart rate monitor can help you become more emotionally, metabolically, and physically fit because it informs you of certain changes taking place in your body. It tells you how hard you are exercising, reveals the state of your emotions, and helps you determine your energy expenditure. It pulls these physiological variables together, weighs them, and comes up with a signal that reports your overall condition—that is, your heart rate. I'm sure it will join the bathroom scales, the thermometer, and the wristwatch as an essential personal device. Heart rate monitors don't cost much. You can easily obtain one. They deliver accurate readings. They are easy and fun to use, and they motivate you.

Trust me. Get a heart monitor. When you do, you'll wonder how you lived without it and its reliable translation of the language of your heart. You'll start using it slowly, capturing a single number such as your resting heart rate. Then, as you learn of the language of your heart, you will place that number in context with other numbers that will open up a whole new world of fitness for you, just as it did for Mike.

What Can a Heart Rate Monitor Do?

Your workouts will be more effective, efficient, and full if you base them on the amount of physical effort rather than distance or time. A heart rate monitor is the only way you can accurately measure the degree of physical effort, or load, without an entourage of exercise scientists following your every move. The heart rate monitor opens a window into your body's response to the moment-to-moment changes in your physical activity.

A heart rate monitor is actually a number of different tools all rolled into one. It informs you about your fitness, what type of energy you are using, your stress levels, and your emotions. Some health practitioners even use heart rate as a medical test for food intolerance, while forensic specialists use it in lie-detection devices. For athletes, it takes the guesswork out of training. By using the data it provides, you can control your training level and maximize the results from your training.

Here's just a sample of how you can use a heart rate monitor:

- **A fitness monitor.** You can measure your current level of fitness and how much fitter you are becoming as you exercise more. You can optimize your training to ensure that you achieve your goals. What you can measure, you can manipulate more accurately. Take the guesswork out of exercise and take a shortcut to success that guarantees more benefits in less time.

- **A fuel gauge.** Knowing your heart rate boundaries and using them to measure and manipulate your exercise intensities helps you to understand whether you are burning mostly fat or mostly carbohydrate, how fast you are burning up your energy reserves, and when you could run out.

- **A stress monitor.** The monitor never lies. If you wear your monitor while driving your car in rush hour traffic, you'll see the actual physical effects of the stress caused by bumper-to-bumper congestion. Alton Skinner, who designs fitness programs for golfers and wrote *The Stroke-saver Workout,* instructs his clients to wear a monitor during a round of golf. A neurosurgeon discovered that his heart rate shot up whenever he putted (higher, in fact, than when he performed brain surgery). Alton's clients use this feedback to calm their hearts and lower their scores.

- **An animal-training aid.** Famous horse trainer Monty Roberts uses heart rate to train the handlers of nervous or disobedient horses because that nervousness often results from the handler's nervousness. Horses are extremely sensitive to our physical condition and can sense our elevated heart rates. Monty teaches people to lower their heart rates before inter-acting with the horse, with amazing results. The horse instantly displays greater confidence and trust in the handler. He says the techniques work well with children and teenagers, too.

- **A love monitor.** Slip on your monitor during a passionate moment with a loved one, and observe the effects of joy on your heart. The monitor truly does show the link between your mind and your heart.

- **A motivational tool.** Training with a heart rate monitor is like having a portable fitness coach strapped to your wrist. Whenever you use your monitor as a guide, a friend, a coach, or a training partner, you enjoy a constant companion who understands the language of the heart. Some-times it's hard to maintain your motivation during an exercise program because you don't see any rapid physical changes taking place. These sometimes take several months to appear. However, changes in your heart happen much more rapidly, even over a few weeks. Your monitor will show them to you and thus inspire you to keep going.

What You Can Do with Your Heart Rate Monitor: Lorraine's Story

Lorraine tells us how she's used her heart rate monitor:

I was very excited to receive my first heart rate monitor as a gift. The first thing I wanted to do with it was wear it to bed, but my husband objected: He thought I might try to measure his performance using it!

I used my heart rate monitor to learn to run. At first I ran until I reached a certain heart rate and walked until I recovered again and again until after several weeks I was running longer than walking.

I almost got into trouble with my heart rate monitor at work because a colleague and I were discovered competing to get our heart rates as low as possible during a particularly uninteresting meeting.

I used it to lower my heart rate before an important presentation at work and discovered that it helped get rid of that squeaky voice you get when you get nervous.

Of course, I used my heart rate monitor to train for a triathlon and my first marathon. My greatest source of pride is that I used speed/heart rate measurements to make a race plan that allowed me to complete my first marathon within my planned schedule, without running out of energy, and getting faster over the course of the race.

Right now my heart rate monitor is giving me important information on the changing physiology of my advancing pregnancy. My delta heart rate is high, my recovery heart rate is terrible, and my resting heart rate is increasing as my belly grows. Being able to see the additional work my heart is doing is helping me to accept the increasing physical limitations at this time and make the appropriate modifications to my training and lifestyle.

How to Buy a Heart Rate Monitor

You will find there more than 100 different models on the market today, ranging from the simplest to the most complex, from one that displays only your current heart rate to one that can store information that you can download later into your computer. Different brands and models of heart rate monitors offer a range of features and functions. As a rule, the more functions and features you get, the more you pay. You should consider the following functions and features when shopping for your own monitor.

Type of Transmission

Just like mobile phones, heart rate monitors transmit data from the chest belt to the wrist receiver by either analog radio waves or coded, digital waves. Most devices use the older analog system. However, just like old analog mobile phones, the analog system can be disrupted by interference from other heart rate monitors and electronic equipment. To get around this problem, manufacturers either provide a coded analog transmission, whereby the monitor transmits on 1 of 42 different channels or frequencies, or adopt a digital technology system. You will benefit from coded or digital transmission if you want to use your heart rate monitor in a crowded health club environment.

Watch Functions

As soon as you start to train with your monitor, you will probably appreciate the advantage of more features than simply your heart rate (time of day, a stopwatch, or a light, for example). Some people want to wear their heart rate monitor like a normal watch, and they demand date and alarm features, too. Others want something sleek and fashionable, while still others like a sporty look or large, easy-to-read digits.

Sport Functions

Depending on your choice of sport, you might want sport-specific features, such as a good handlebar mount if you are a cyclist, plus other cycling information like speed, distance, riding time, cadence, and power output. If you swim, you will prefer the most watertight monitor you can get (though you might trade this feature for the ability to change the chest strap battery yourself). Mountaineers enjoy integrated altitude information, while back-country skiers want to see speed of ascent and descent. Multisport athletes look for split timing functions. If you train with a horse, you might want a heart rate monitor for the animal, too. Adventure racers may value ruggedness over all other features.

Training Functions

At first you will use your monitor to gain information about your right-now heart rate, but you might want it to store information about your training session. This could save you having to write down or remember numbers during your workout.

Information useful during training includes the following:

- Whether you are in a particular heart-training zone (either with graphics on the display or an audible alarm, which you can turn on or off)
- Percent of maximum heart rate
- Average heart rate during the workout
- Exercise time and lap or split times (stop watch functions)
- A preprogrammed workout that guides you through your training

Data useful to review later includes the following:

- Time spent in different heart training zones (some monitors give you this information for only one zone, others for all five)
- Exercise and lap or split times
- Peak heart rate
- Average heart rate
- Actual heart rate at different points in your workout (some monitors store your actual heart rate every 5, 13, or 30 seconds, while others do it only when you press the buttons)
- Average and peak heart rates per lap or split
- Estimation of calories used
- Recovery heart rate data

The ability to program the monitor will probably be a valuable feature as you learn more about heart rate monitors. Useful programming features include the following:

- Your own individual maximum heart rate and training zones
- Different maximum heart rate for different sports
- Adaptation to different users
- Different time zones
- Customized display to show only relevant training information

Data Storage

Different heart rate monitors store different amounts of information. Some just tell you what's happening while you are exercising; some save it so that you can look at the data afterward. The latter will appeal to you if you want to track your progress over time. Ask these questions:

- How long are my workouts?
- Will the watch hold all my information?
- Do I want to do multiple workouts before I look at the data?
- Can I adjust the recording interval and thereby extend the memory of the monitor?
- Which data is stored for later recall, and which is displayed only at the moment?

Data Recall

Data recall features also vary from monitor to monitor. Some allow you to read the data off the monitor display, while others permit you to download the information into your personal computer. Downloadable monitors cost a lot more, but they do let you see your heart rate for your entire workout, store key training information, track your training intensity, and analyze your performance and improvement over time. The different types of downloading methods include the following:

- **Manual recall.** Scrolling data on the monitor display.

- **Infrared.** Direct data transfer via infrared radio waves from the monitor into your computer. If you don't have an infrared port, you must purchase a special interface to accomplish this.

- **Sonic transfer.** Direct data transfer via audible radio waves from the monitor into the computer via the computer's microphone.

- **Manufacturer's interface.** Direct data transfer from the monitor into the computer via a special interface box supplied by the heart rate monitor manufacturer.

Software Functions

Downloadable heart rate monitors are normally sold with a proprietary software program. You can also obtain other software that can help you manipulate the data. Useful features in these programs allow you to ...

- Add supplementary information about your training.

- Include daily information, such as weight, sleep quality, and weather conditions.

- Analyze workouts.

- Export data to other software programs.

Gimmicks

In addition to all sorts of useful features, some heart rate monitors offer some gimmicks that don't actually help you train and can confuse you with irrelevant information. Some of these functions can actually mislead you, make the heart rate monitor more difficult to operate, and distract you from recognizing useful features when making a purchase. Some gimmicky functions that you might find not so useful when you actually start training with your heart rate monitor are discussed next.

Calculation of Maximum Heart Rate

Some heart rate monitors promise to calculate your maximum heart rate for you. They base this calculation on such information as your age, physical condition, and weight. Sometimes they require you to perform a standard test protocol before estimating your maximum heart rate. These monitors rely on standard equations programmed into them. However, your maximum heart rate is unique. Thus, the best way to find out your own maximum heart rate involves testing it yourself using one or several of the methods described in this book. Make sure you can manually enter your own individually tested maximum heart rate into the monitor.

Fitness Tests

Some heart rate monitors offer tests, claiming to measure your level of aerobic fitness from your resting heart rate over a five-minute period. They derive these tests from the relationship between aerobic fitness and heart rate variability (the degree to which the shape of your heart beat waves vary between beats). Although ingenious, these tests depend on averaged census data and cannot match simple tests you can perform manually.

Calculation of Heart Training Zones

Some heart rate monitors can calculate and set up your heart-training zones for you. If you are considering purchasing one that does this, make sure it sets up the zones the way you prefer. For instance, are there three or five zones, how are they set, and can you change them?

No Chest Strap Required

Some heart rate monitors can operate without a chest strap. While things may change as technology progresses, at the moment strapless chest monitors do not offer continuous heart rate data (you must stop and press your fingers on the monitor and wait for your heart rate to appear). Because your heart rate drops when you stop to take a reading, you will always get a more accurate reading with a monitor that gives you a continuous heart rate reading, which currently can't be achieved without the use of a chest strap.

Estimation of Proportion of Calories Used as Fat

Although you do want to gain an appreciation of the types of fuel you burn when you exercise, any data provided to you via a heart rate monitor will most likely be so general that it is virtually useless. The proportion of fuels you use at different exercise intensities varies according to many factors, including your current level of fitness, your diet, what you just ate, how long you exercise, the temperature, and many other factors. No monitor can yet take all these variables into account—at least, not accurately.

Fat Trap: Heart Rate Monitors and Calorie Use

Some monitors estimate how many calories you use as you exercise. The monitor calculates your calorie expenditure based on your heart rate and your weight, assuming that the harder you exercise and the more you weigh, the more calories you will burn (based on standard equations obtained from measurements of a large number of people).

That's useful data, but you should bear in mind that the calculation may be quite inaccurate. The actual relationship between energy expenditure and heart rate is highly individual and will vary depending on the type of activity. For example, during weight training your heart rate may not climb above 120 bpm, yet you could be expending far more energy than walking fast at the same rate. Therefore, estimates can mislead you.

You must place such data in the context of your particular type of workout. If you swim for one hour and, according to your heart rate monitor, burn 500 calories, that session wasn't as hard as one in which you swam more vigorously for one hour and, according to the same monitor, burned 800 calories. Never forget that you must treat yourself (and your exercise program) as the unique individual you are.

Using a Heart Rate Monitor

When you turn on any heart rate monitor, ignore the first few numbers that appear because the software requires several sample heart rates before it can calculate an accurate number. Likewise, if you quickly increase your heart rate, the heart rate values on your monitor lag behind your real heart rate number because of the time it takes for the device's software to average the data.

If you don't buy or borrow a monitor or find one built into a piece of exercise equipment, such as a treadmill, you can still do all of the following activities by manually counting your heart rate for 6 seconds and multiplying the result by 10. Though this is not as convenient or quick, it still gives numbers that you can use. However, from this point on, all activities and workouts in this book involving heart rate will assume you are using a heart rate monitor.

Activity 3.1: Getting Acquainted with Your Heart Rate Monitor

You're ready to start using the language of the heart to begin designing your unique training program. For your first experience, read the user's manual that comes with the monitor and learn how to wear it and program it. Try wearing it during normal activities for a day or two. You'll probably get some surprises, such as how little or how much a given activity raises your heart rate.

As you go about your daily activities, glance at your monitor to get a feel for how your heart is working while you're walking, gardening, or playing tennis. When do you see the lowest numbers? When do you see the highest numbers? What effects does a given activity have on your heart rate?

Write down in your logbook a list of your daily routines and the heart rates associated with them. For example, Lorraine wrote down the following list after wearing her heart rate monitor for one week.

Lorraine's Daily Activity Heart Rate Log

Waking heart rate	72
Midmorning heart rate at work	64
Midafternoon heart rate at work	58
Cycling to work	120 to 130
Making a telephone call at work	85 to 95
Climbing the 104 stairs to her apartment	155
During long afternoon meetings	52

The Snowflake Principle

No two snowflakes are identical. Nor are any two people. So why would anyone follow a fitness program designed for the so-called "average" person? Celebrities promote their proven programs, authors tout their patented workouts or diets, and athletes show the secrets of their success. In reality, there is no such thing as a one-size-fits-all program.

Oh, all those books, articles, websites, and speakers advising you to buy into their programs mean well. And I'm sure many people have benefited from these best-sellers, but you'll gain so much more from a program you build around your own body, heart, dreams, and lifestyle. All metabolic, emotional, and physical fitness plans must accommodate one undeniable, irrevocable, unarguable law: We are all different. Just as every snowflake's pattern is unique to it, one of the smallest components of life, your DNA, is unique to you. Furthermore, your fitness program must also progress with you, at your pace, in the direction you want it to go and in a way that fits your life. Your heart rate monitor gives you some of the vital information you need to follow that rule.

Each of us possesses our own unique biological makeup. Our physiology and biology, all the cells of our bodies, and their functions differ. So do our body types, stages in life, ages, sports and fitness backgrounds, skill sets, muscle types, environmental influences, goals, preferences, competitiveness, biomechanics, injuries, and levels of enjoyment playing or working at various intensities, frequencies, and duration. When you start your training program, remember that it needs to fit you: your schedule, your interests, and your unique biological makeup.

Now that you've determined your resting, delta, and recovery heart rates, the next step is to find your maximum heart rate: the maximum number of times your heart can beat in one minute. You were born with this unique number, which doesn't change throughout your entire life (although your ability to achieve it may decrease if you become unfit). A relatively high maximum heart rate doesn't confer any athletic advantage on a person, nor does a relatively low one signal a problem; it's just a number. But it does tell you something important: the upper limit for how fast your heart can go—a limit you will use to establish the training intensities in your fitness program. It's a key physiological anchor point, a point of reference for gauging your level of intensity during exercise.

The only other reliable anchor point is your VO_2 max (maximum volume of oxygen consumption), or the ability of your cardiovascular system to deliver oxygen to the muscles. Determining that number, however, requires hooking yourself up to a breath analyzer in a laboratory, which is not something convenient for every workout.

You may have heard that the way you calculate your maximum heart rate is to use a formula such as 220 minus your age. In fact, William Haskell, Ph.D., who originally developed the formula in the early 1970s, never intended it to be an absolute guide to training. He knew that the study group was not representative of the general population and that normal people could experience a 20-beat variation in their actual maximum heart rate, as compared to their predicted maximum heart rate using the equation[1]. Recently, researchers at the University of New Mexico, Albuquerque, reviewed the development of the equation and data from more recent studies and firmly concluded that "the formula 220 – age has no scientific merit for use in exercise physiology and related fields."[2] They found that the most accurate general equation, if you must use one, is this:

Predicted maximum heart rate = 205.8 – 0.685 (age)

Even so, there could be a six-beat error.

The most reliable way you can find your maximum heart rate is to test it. A full maximum heart rate test takes your heart to the maximum level and is specifically designed to stress the body to its limit. You might not be ready for this; in this case, you might not want to try a full maximum heart rate test until you become fully accustomed to hard exercise. If you do want the full test, consult Appendix B. A less strenuous, albeit somewhat less accurate, approach is to take a series of submaximum tests:

- Setting your peak heart rate number (Activity 3.2)
- Doing the one-mile walk heart rate test (Activity 3.3)
- Doing the step heart rate test (Activity 3.4)

Averaged together, along with a mathematical calculation of your maximum heart rate (Activity 3.5), the following three submaximum tests will give you a reasonably accurate maximum heart rate estimate. Activity 3.6 will guide you through the calculations to find your maximum heart rate.

Activity 3.2: Setting Your Peak Heart Rate Number

Your peak heart rate is the highest number you can get on your heart rate monitor while exercising as hard as you can. Though it is below your maximum heart rate, it comes close enough to be useful.

If you swim or bike or walk, do it as strenuously as you can. Then record the highest number you see in your personal fitness log.

My peak heart rate number is: _____ bpm

Activity 3.3: One-Mile Walking Heart Rate Number

Go to any high school or college track (most are 400 meters or 440 yards around), and walk or stride as fast as you comfortably can in your current condition. Walk four continuous laps. On the last lap, take your pulse or use your heart rate monitor to determine your average heart rate for *only* that lap. The first three laps just get you to a heart rate plateau where you'll stay for the last lap.

My one-mile walk heart rate number is: _____ bpm

Activity 3.4: The Step Heart Rate Number

Using an eight-inch step (almost any step in your home or in a club will do), you can perform a three-minute step test. After you warm up with a short walk or by stretching, step up and down in a four-count sequence as follows: right foot up, left foot up, right foot down, left foot down. Each time you move a foot up or down, it counts as one step. Count "up, up, down, down" for 1 set, with 20 sets to the minute. Don't speed up the pace—keep it regular. Determine your average heart rate for the last one minute of this three-minute exercise period.

My three-minute step heart rate number is: _____ bpm

Activity 3.5: The Math Max Heart Rate Number

You can also estimate your maximum heart rate with this math equation:

Predicted maximum heart rate = 205.8 − 0.685 (age)

For example, here's how Mike calculated his:

205.8 − 0.685 (54) = 168.81 bpm

My math max heart rate number is: _____ bpm

Activity 3.6: Submax (Submaximum) Results

These four activities should give you a fairly accurate measurement of your maximum heart rate. That number, an important part of your biological makeup, will enable you to determine each of the five different fitness-training intensities we'll discuss in a moment. Average the five numbers you obtained, using the form below, and then use the result as your estimated maximum heart rate.

Calculation of Estimated Maximum Heart Rate

My peak heart rate number is:	_____ bpm
My one-mile walk heart rate number is:	_____ bpm
My three-minute step heart rate number is:	_____ bpm
My math max heart rate number is:	_____ bpm
Total =	_____ bpm
Average (÷ 4) =	_____ bpm

Assessing Your Current Level of Fitness

Before you launch your program based on the calculation of your estimated maximum heart rate, pause for a moment to classify your current level of fitness. Select the category you feel best represents your current level:

- **Poor shape.** You do not exercise at all and are sedentary, or you have not exercised in the last six to eight weeks. Remember, you can be thin and still be in poor shape.

- **Average shape.** You walk a mile 3 times a week, or you participate in any aerobic activity 3 times a week for 20 minutes. You have completed one to three hours of physical training per week for the past six to eight weeks.

- **Excellent shape.** You regularly do cardiovascular training sessions that together total more than three to five hours a week, or you walk or run at least five miles a week.

- **Athletic shape.** You are in great cardiovascular shape and have been working out more than five hours a week for six months to a year, and you enjoy participating in events such as runs, walks, cycling, and triathlons.

You can now refine your estimated maximum heart rate by incorporating your current level of fitness into your calculations. Put your results from the submax tests in Column A, and then add the appropriate fitness factor in Column B to your one-mile walking heart rate and to your three-minute step heart rate. Add columns A and B together, and then average the results to get a more accurate estimate of your maximum heart rate.

Refining Your Estimated Maximum Heart Rate

Fit *and* Fat Activity	Heart Rate Result (A)	Fitness Factor (B)	Estimated Maximum Heart Rate (A+B)
Peak heart rate	_____ bpm	Nothing to add	_____ bpm
One-mile walking heart rate	_____ bpm	Poor + 40 bpm Average + 50 bpm Excellent + 60 bpm Athletic + 70 bpm	_____ bpm

Refining Your Estimated Maximum Heart Rate *continued*

Fit *and* Fat Activity	Heart Rate Result (A)	Fitness Factor (B)	Estimated Maximum Heart Rate (A+B)
Three-minute step heart rate	_____ bpm	Poor + 55 bpm Average + 65 bpm Excellent + 75 bpm Athletic + 85 bpm	_____ bpm
Math max heart rate	_____ bpm	Nothing to add	_____ bpm
		Total number:	_____
		Divide by 4:	_____
		Estimated maximum heart rate:	_____ bpm

Introducing the Five Heart Zones

In the old days, advice on physical conditioning amounted to something like "Figure out what 60 percent to 80 percent of your maximum heart rate is, using the equation 220 – age, and go train in this 'target zone' for 30 minutes 5 times a week." Well, unfortunately, it's not quite as simple as this. Fortunately, you don't have to waste your time trying a one-size-fits-all exercise program that may or may not work for you. This is because not all exercise is equal. What happens to your body when you train at a heart rate of 50 to 60 percent of your maximum heart rate is entirely different from what happens when you train at 80 to 90 percent of your maximum heart rate.

To give you a framework to structure your training, I developed a system of training that involves not just one, but five heart zones. Each zone is 10 percent of your maximum heart rate, starting at 50 percent. Why start at 50 percent of the maximum heart rate? Well, that's the exercise intensity at which most of us start to notice the effort of training and at which we start to get benefits from our effort. Each of the five heart zone training zones feels different, stimulates different aspects of our fitness during our training, uses different energy systems, and results in different health benefits after the training. The features and benefits of the five zones are summarized in the following table. In general, the lower zones provide general health and wellness benefits, including metabolic and emotional fitness benefits, and the higher zones offer more performance-type improvements to your fitness.

The benefits of each zone are specific to that zone, not cumulative. This means that you get the benefits of Zone 1 only when you train in that zone. The zones are also synergistic. This means that the value of training in one zone one day is amplified by training the next day in a different zone. To receive a full spectrum of health and fitness rewards, you need to train in the full spectrum of zones. No one zone is the ideal training zone with the greatest bang for your buck: You will need all zones to get a full range of benefits.

The Five Heart Zones

Heart Zone	Description	Activity
Zone 1, The Healthy Heart Zone	This is a low-intensity heart zone where you work out at 50 to 60 percent of your maximum heart rate.	Spending time in this heart zone results in measurable metabolic improvement, enhanced self-esteem, improved blood chemistry, and stabilization of body weight gains.
Zone 2, The Temperate Zone	This is a moderate-intensity heart zone where you work out at 60 to 70 percent of your maximum heart rate.	Spending time in this heart zone results in improved energy metabolism, increased number of total and fat calories burned, and enhancement of cardiovascular endurance.
Zone 3, The Aerobic Zone	This is a more intense heart zone where you work out at 70 to 80 percent of your maximum heart rate.	Spending time in this heart zone results in measurable improvements in your oxygen-carrying (aerobic) capacity, improved muscle power, and increases in fat burning.
Zone 4, The Threshold Zone	This is a very intense training zone where you work out at 80 to 90 percent of your maximum heart rate.	This represents a shift to changes that improve sports performance. Also known as the Threshold Zone to represent the shift toward carbohydrate metabolism.
Zone 5, The Red Line Zone	This is the toughest zone where you work out at 90 to 100 percent of your maximum heart rate.	Like its name, this zone is high, hot, and hard. This is all-out effort; you are most prone to injury in this zone.

69

Activity 3.7: Setting Your Heart Zones

Now that you have pinpointed your estimated maximum heart rate, you can set your target training zones with the heart zones chart. A heart zone is a range of heart beats, each a percentage of your maximum heart rate, that deliver different physical, emotional, and metabolic fitness benefits. To obtain the most benefits from your training program, you will want to spend time in all five zones.

Training Zone (% maximum heart rate)	Fuel Burning	M A X I M U M H E A R T R A T E													
		Max HR 150	Max HR 155	Max HR 160	Max HR 165	Max HR 170	Max HR 175	Max HR 180	Max HR 185	Max HR 190	Max HR 195	Max HR 200	Max HR 205	Max HR 210	Max HR 215	Max HR 220
Z5 RED LINE 90%-100%	GLYCOGEN BURNING	135	140	144	149	153	158	162	167	171	176	180	185	189	194	198
Z4 THRESHOLD 80%-90%		135–120	140–124	144–128	149–132	153–136	158–140	162–144	167–148	171–152	176–156	180–160	185–164	189–168	194–172	198–176
Z3 AEROBIC 70%-80%		120–105	124–109	128–112	132–116	136–119	140–123	144–126	148–130	152–133	156–137	160–140	164–144	168–147	172–151	176–154
Z2 TEMPERATE 60%-70%	FAT BURNING	105–90	109–93	112–96	116–99	119–102	123–105	126–108	130–111	133–114	137–117	140–120	144–123	147–126	151–129	154–132
Z1 HEALTHY HEART 50%-60%		90–75	93–78	96–80	99–83	102–85	105–88	108–90	111–93	114–95	117–98	120–100	123–103	126–105	129–108	132–110

The Heart Zones. Read your estimated maximum heart rate along the top and then read down to find your five Heart Zones.

Instead of calculating your individual heart zones, you can find them from the preceding figure. To find the ceiling and the floor for each of your five heart zones, circle the number on the top column that is closest to your estimated maximum heart rate; then read down the column to read off the upper (ceiling) and lower (floor) limits of each zone. Write down your heart rate numbers for each of the five zones. You will need these important numbers in your training.

My Heart Zones

Zone	Floor	Ceiling
Zone 1 (50 to 60 percent)	_____	_____
Zone 2 (60 to 70 percent)	_____	_____
Zone 3 (70 to 80 percent)	_____	_____
Zone 4 (80 to 90 percent	_____	_____
Zone 5 (90 to 100 percent)	_____	_____

Activity 3.8: The Four-Minute Tour de Zones

Now that you have set your particular heart rate zones, you are ready to get acquainted with the first three: zones 1, 2, and 3. Even if you are an experienced exerciser, you should complete this workout. As you spend time in each zone, try to feel their individual characteristics. You should notice a fairly dramatic difference between Zone 1 (50 to 60 percent maximum heart rate) and Zone 3 (70 to 80 percent maximum heart rate).

Touring the three lower zones, the health and fitness zones, provides an excellent experience with varying exercise intensity. At different levels of intensity in the various zones, different things happen inside your body, producing different results.

To do the workout, choose a training mode—for example, walking/running, swimming, biking, rowing, stepping—that will enable you to reach zones 1 through 3 (50 to 75 percent of your maximum heart rate). Let's use walking as an example:

1. You'll warm up for a few minutes, stretching your leg muscles and walking at a leisurely pace. Then you'll intensify your effort until you reach 50 percent of your maximum heart rate. For example, with a maximum heart rate of 169, Mike walks leisurely for a quarter of a mile before his monitor reaches 89.

2. Whatever exercise you choose should allow you to maintain 50 to 60 percent (Zone 1) of your maximum heart rate for four minutes.

3. Then increase the intensity of your workout until you reach Zone 2 (60 to 70 percent). A quarter mile farther into his walk, for example, Mike reaches 115 bpm. Once again, stay in Zone 2 for four minutes.

4. At the end of four minutes, push yourself into Zone 3. At about three quarters of a mile, Mike hits 75 percent of his maximum heart rate (127 bpm). He's walking quite fast at this point, bunking into a light jog. He's feeling it: He's sweating, his muscles begin to tire a bit, his heart is racing, and he's breathing hard. Stay in Zone 3 for four minutes.

5. Now you reverse the process, dropping into Zone 2 for four minutes.

6. Then drop into Zone 1 for four minutes.

7. Finally, you should cool yourself down so that your heart rate drops below 100.

This whole workout will take you 26 minutes to complete.

71

Activity 3.8. *continued*

Training in the low zones will improve your metabolic fitness. Spending time in them results in improvements in blood pressure, body weight, and cholesterol levels. It also reduces emotional stress and leads to more energy. Enjoy the four-minute drill. I sure do. Use the following workout plan to guide you through the workout. A blank workout form is provided in Appendix F for you to fill in your own heart rate numbers.

Four-Minute Tour de Zones Workout

Elapsed Time (Min)	Workout Plan	Heart Zone	Your Heart Rate (bpm)	Interval Time (Min)
0 to 4	Warm up in Zone 1	1	_____	4
4 to 8	Increase HR to middle of Zone 2	2	_____	4
8 to 12	Increase HR to middle of Zone 3	3	_____	4
12 to 16	Decrease HR to middle of Zone 2	2	_____	4
16 to 22	Decrease HR to middle of Zone 1	1	_____	4
22 to 26	Cool down to below 100 bpm	<1	_____	6

The following figure shows you what your heart rate would look like if you plotted it on a graph through the workout.

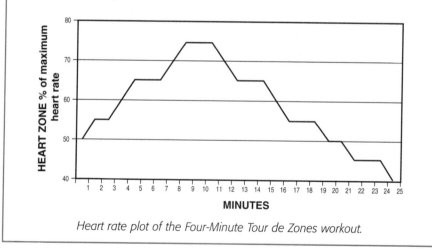

Heart rate plot of the Four-Minute Tour de Zones workout.

Tailor the Workout to Your Fitness Level

All workouts should suit your individual, unique, and personal physiology. If you have just begun fitness training, modify the Four-Minute Tour de Zones workout by decreasing the amount of time spent in each zone by one minute. If you are super fit, increase the time in each zone by two minutes and double up in Zone 3. The modified workout plans are shown in the following table.

Four-Minute Tour de Zones Workout, Modified for Beginners

Elapsed Time (Min)	Workout Plan	Heart Zone	Your Heart Rate (bpm)	Interval Time (Min)
0 to 3	Warm up in Zone 1	1	_____	3
3 to 6	Increase HR to middle of Zone 2	2	_____	3
6 to 9	Increase HR to middle of Zone 3	3	_____	3
9 to 12	Decrease HR to middle of Zone 2	2	_____	3
12 to 15	Decrease HR to middle of Zone 1	1	_____	3
15 to 18	Cool down to below 100 bpm	<1	_____	3

Four-Minute Tour de Zones Workout, Modified for Advanced Level

Elapsed Time (Min)	Workout Plan	Heart Zone	Your Heart Rate (bpm)	Interval Time (Min)
0 to 6	Warm up in Zone 1	1	_____	6
6 to 12	Increase HR to middle of Zone 2	2	_____	6
12 to 20	Increase HR to middle of Zone 3	3	_____	8
20 to 26	Decrease HR to middle of Zone 2	2	_____	6
26 to 32	Decrease HR to middle of Zone 1	1	_____	6
32 to 38	Cool down to below 100 bpm	<1	_____	6

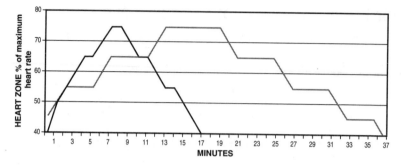

Heart rate plot of the Four-Minute Tour de Zones workout, modified for Beginner and Advanced Levels.

Week 2 Summary

During this week, you started to learn the language of the heart. You began to appreciate the value of using a heart rate monitor to get the information you need to launch yourself on the path to greater fitness. With it, you established your maximum heart rate and set up your zones. Your first heart zones workout gave you a feeling for how your body reacts in zones 1, 2, and 3. Congratulations! You've found the path to becoming an athlete. Maintain the changes you made this week, and note improvements in your emotions, your attitudes, and the way you feel in your personal fitness log.

CHAPTER 4

Week 3: Energywise
Achieving Your Own Best Balance

Fat is in your body, not your head. Bonnie Cook made legal history in 1993. She had applied for work at a home for the mentally disadvantaged, where she had previously worked between 1978 and 1980, and 1981 to 1986. On both occasions, she left voluntarily under good terms with her employer, the Rhode Island Department of Mental Health, Retardation, and Hospitals. However, this time she had put on a lot of weight: At 5 feet, 2 inches and 320 pounds, she was more than double her ideal body weight for her height and was clinically obese. The doctor responsible for approving her employment application rejected it, saying that her weight gain had compromised her ability to carry out her duties and had also increased her risk of heart disease, making her more likely to need worker's compensation at some point in the future. Shocked by the rejection, Bonnie sued Rhode Island State, under the Rehabilitation Act and the Americans with Disabilities Act, for discriminating against her on account of her fitness. She insisted that she could carry out her job just as well as she had before. She won the suit and was awarded $100,000 and the right to the next available and suitable position at the institute.

Why did she prevail? The lawyer presenting Bonnie's case, Lynette Labinger, invited a medical expert on obesity to testify on Bonnie's behalf. Arthur Frank, M.D., the Medical Director of the George Washington University Obesity Management Program, spoke very simply to the court. He began by using himself as an example, telling the jury that he was what he called a "random eater." He went on, "I don't pay any attention to what I eat, and over the last 20 years my weight hasn't changed at all." He then explained to the court how little beyond his required intake of calories he would have to eat to gain weight: Just an extra two to three peanuts a day could cause him to gain a pound a year. Knowing that this just didn't happen to most adult humans, he explained that one must logically conclude that our bodies take care of our weight without any conscious effort.

In a peer-reviewed article in the *Journal of the American Medical Association*,[1] Frank had written that "nature does not permit body weight to fluctuate randomly in other mammals" and that "it is inconceivable that humans would have a randomly unstable weight ...." Furthermore, he said, "even obese people are usually weight stable." Frank explained that the body normally defends weight loss or gain through powerful regulatory mechanisms and that, despite the fact we can sometimes override these mechanisms through deliberate effort or because of a change in the emotional climate, "there is no reason to believe that patient's behavior causes [obesity]."

Frank's argument broke from the conventional wisdom of the time, which insisted that fat people lacked self-control and brought their condition upon themselves. The conventional view created a huge burden of guilt for fat people, a condition as worrisome to their health as the extra fat they already carried. To the contrary, Frank argued, some people are susceptible to weight gain because their bodies do not defend the "ideal weight" in the way those of lean people do. For a person susceptible to weight gain and subject to the type of environment that allows weight gain to happen (one of high food availability coupled with a lack of physical activity), obesity is not a psychological phenomenon. It's a biochemical one.

Labinger used Frank's testimony to argue that Bonnie was not the victim of her own poor choices and overindulgences, but the victim of a biochemical makeup that she could not completely control. The jury agreed. And so should you. Fatness does not occur because of psychological deficiencies or behavioral defects. It is a complex process involving many biological variables scientists have only just begun to understand. Sometimes, despite rigorous self-control and admirable eating habits, we remain powerless to manage our weight. Our stubborn bodies like to manage their own weight and don't always obey our wishes. Thus, it makes sense that we should strive to understand some of the processes involved in the complex mechanism of weight regulation. If we could gain a better understanding of how our bodies work, we would give ourselves the opportunity to do something that helps them to work in a way that awards better health and well-being. During this week, you'll learn about how to find your own best balance.

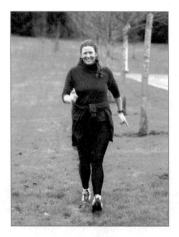

Marry Clayton enjoying a run to stay fit and healthy.

It's Not All About What You Put in Your Mouth

You're probably wondering, "What about eating? What exactly should I eat?" Good question. No health and fitness program would be complete without some advice on eating. By this point, however, you know that, for almost all people, lack of exercise accounts for the trend toward fat more than food, and that how much we move deserves more attention than what we eat. Researchers have already recognized that when you lead an active life, you can more easily and naturally attain a steady weight. That's how I live: getting the exercise I need for my body to remain healthy and eating what my body tells me I need. I want you to live like that, too, getting in touch with the miraculous way the human body tells when it's hungry, thirsty, full, or overfed, and when it needs different types of nutrients.

The food industry encourages us to eat ever larger portions[2] and more calorie-dense foods, which ends up driving the diet industry and, in turn, maintains our focus on food. Now researchers are beginning to realize that it's not simply what we put in our mouths, but, more important, how our bodies deal with what we eat and how much activity we require of our bodies. An old cliché proposes: *You are what you eat.* However, my personal experience and intensive research convinces me that you are what you *do*. Or put another way, you are the sum total of your physical, emotional, and metabolic fitness. Scientists have only begun to figure out how the body balances energy and the complex ways in which our daily environment affects the body's ability to do this well. Nevertheless, we do know this: The body's ability to balance energy can be compromised either by something within us that gets out of sync or by an unsuitable environment.

It happened to Ann, who bore her first child in her mid-30s. It was a difficult pregnancy from the start and ended with a traumatic emergency cesarean and, to Ann's ultimate relief, a wonderful baby girl, Hannah. Ann and her husband grow their own produce, collect wild foods, and make just about everything they eat the old-fashioned way. Combined with an outdoor lifestyle and a love of cycling, Ann's way of living had always enabled her to maintain a healthy weight and plenty of vitality. But her life after Hannah's birth brought unexpected changes. The weight she had gained in pregnancy would not go away—worse, more kept piling on. When Ann looked closely at her eating habits, her emotional state, and her exercise routine, she couldn't understand why what had worked before childbirth was failing her now. Somehow, her body, the way it worked, the way it grabbed and stored energy, and the way it formerly balanced energy had altered, and weight gain was one of the consequences.

Ann's friend Tina went through a very different life change when she had a hysterectomy in her early 40s. She had always been athletic, climbing mountains on weekends and joining expeditions to explore the Alps, the Rockies, and the Himalayas on holidays. Yes, she had a sweet tooth, but what with a daily routine of walking the dog, gardening, and just living an active lifestyle, she didn't have a problem balancing her energy and maintaining a healthy weight (except maybe at Christmas!). However, after the operation, she quickly gained a tremendous amount of weight. The old strategies she relied on to get back into shape after an overindulgent holiday season no longer worked. Even calorie-controlled diets didn't make a dent in her weight because she always put on even more pounds after the diet. Nothing else had changed or shifted in Tina's lifestyle—not her activity, or her home life, or her job, or even her dog's weight. No, something in Tina's energy-balancing processes had become stuck; something had shifted within her body to cause these sensitive mechanisms to fall out of sync.

Sometimes environmental factors can cause a similar shifting of energy. We accept that certain plants thrive best when in a certain type of soil and climate, that tropical fish require different conditions than trout, and that a Husky dog's physiology will mean that it wilts in Mexico while a Whippet's causes it to suffer in Alaska. We forget that some of us don't thrive in certain environments, most notably those characterized by an overabundance of food and an underabundance of exercise.

For Kevin, the shift occurred when he started a new job that took him to an entirely new environment, offshore on oil and gas platforms in the Gulf of Mexico. It was a unique environment, a bit like living on a ship: The platform moves with the waves, foul weather keeps you inside, and you inhabit a cramped space. It all adds up to an underabundance of exercise opportunities. The platform's kitchen (the galley) stays open around the clock. It's like living on a ship with a 24-hour restaurant on board: an overabundance of food. It's a stressful environment. On the platform, you work hard, often in irregular shifts, for up to one month of offshore duty. It's unpleasant and tough, so the employers try to make it more bearable by providing the best food they can under the conditions. This environment threw Kevin's body out of sync. The galley became a focal point, not only a place to eat, but also a place to socialize with fellow workers. Not surprisingly, Kevin soon found he needed new work clothes a size larger.

Louise and Richard found themselves in a similar predicament when they moved to a new country. Louise and Richard work for a large multinational company that moved them from their home in the Netherlands to Azerbaijan, a former Soviet republic on the coast of the Caspian Sea. There they encountered vastly different opportunities for food and for exercise. The Azerbaijan culture required Louise to go to the market to buy fresh food. If you wanted meat, for example, you visited the butcher, pointed to a live chicken, and asked him for the breast and thighs. Then the butcher took the squawking bird backstage, slaughtered it, carved the ordered pieces, and handed them to you. Louise then needed to store the meat in her refrigerator for at least 24 hours before using it. Unaccustomed to all this, Louise found it hard to stomach. The alternative? Go out to one of the many inexpensive restaurants and avoid all the hassle.

As for exercise, Louise went everywhere by car, often with a driver, for security reasons. At home in the Netherlands she would have bicycled everywhere. She also missed the fields of tulips, where she had loved to cycle on the weekends. After two years, both Louise and Richard had put on a lot of weight in their new environment. The story ends happily, though: As soon as they returned to Europe, they both naturally got back to their normal healthy weights.

Activity 4.1: Recalling Your Natural Balance

If you have struggled with weight issues, think back over different periods of your life. Were there any periods in your life when you didn't worry about weight, when fatness wasn't an issue for you? Can you recall a time when you maintained a stable weight without consciously trying to do so? Think about those times. Write them in your personal fitness log, leaving a space between each period. Now think back to what was happening in your life at that time. How old were you? What was your emotional life like? Did you go to work in an office? Were you going to school or working at home? Can you remember a typical day or week's physical activity? Did you feel healthy? Happy? How would you describe your relationships? Try to identify specific things in your life then that differ from those in your life now. Do you see anything that may have contributed to you having more of a natural balance in the past? To an imbalance today? Note these items in your personal fitness log.

When your body functions efficiently, you revel in your vitality, your health, and your lust for life. Do you feel that way now, or do you feel sluggish and energy-deficient? Your daily level of energy reflects your overall well-being, the meshing of your physical, emotional, and metabolic fitness. This incredible lust for life energy comes from a healthy mind and a healthy body. Whatever you call it (zip, zest, get-up-and-go), its presence signals fitness; its absence signals a lack of fitness, whether metabolic, emotional, or physical. Use Activity 4.2 to think about your how your energy is right now in your life.

Activity 4.2: Rating Your Energy Level

Answer the following questions about your energy levels and write the answers in your personal fitness log.

1. Do you often have to drag yourself out of bed in the morning?

2. Do you suffer a "midafternoon low" feeling and must reach for something sweet or caffeine-laden to keep you going?

3. Do you sometimes plan activities for the evening but then come home from work completely drained and do nothing?

4. Do you often feel so tired that you can't prepare a meal and choose a frozen dinner or a fast-food meal instead?

5. Do you sometimes feel that you can't function without your morning coffee, cigarette, or evening glass of wine?

If you've answered Yes to more than two of these questions, your energy rating is probably low.

Balancing Act

In Chapter 2, you saw how the old way of thinking about health and fitness concentrated on weight. The less you weighed, the healthier you were. The thinner you looked, the fitter you must have been. According to this mentality, the healthiest body looks the leanest. As we now know, this is false logic; that's simply not how the body works, and what really matters is our health.

Trying to achieve thinness—and, thereby, health—by balancing your energy intake with your expenditure of calories seemed so logical 10 years ago. In fact, I myself found it so compelling that I wrote a book in 1988 called *The Equilibrium Plan*. Today I know I was wrong. The equilibrium equation is just nonsense. Now I'm determined to correct my mistake. The pace of new information and the latest research excites me so much because it all reveals an important truth: You *can* be fit *and* fat.

Let's look more closely at the flaw in the old logic. It stated, via a simple Energy Equation, that if you consume more calories than you use, you gain weight. If you create a deficit of calories by dieting or increasing your physical activity, you lose weight. Here's an example of how the logic worked. Suppose that each day for a year you eat one candy bar more than your energy requirements. The simple math of the Energy Equation allows us to calculate the weight gain that would result from such a modest overindulgence:

Eat one candy bar, which contains 230 calories, every day for a year, and you should theoretically gain 24 pounds. It's easy math:

365 days × 1 candy bar (230 calories) = 83,950 calories

1 pound of fat is equal to 3,500 calories

83,950 divided by 3,500 = 24 pounds of fat

Scary, isn't it? The Energy Equation tells us that if we get the balance of energy just a little bit wrong and make just a small error, dire consequences will follow. But we know that such a scenario just doesn't happen in the real world.

Trust me. The body's feedback system, its management controls, and other dynamic mechanisms disallow the physical laws of simple Energy Equations from applying in a mathematical way. By way of illustration, take a middle-aged man requiring 2,000 calories per day. If over a 10-year period the man gains 5 pounds, we can calculate the difference between calorie input and output over that time period at a mere $^2/_{10}$ of 1 percent:

2,000 calories per day × 365 days × 10 years = 7,300,000 calories

5 pounds = 3,500 calories × 5 = 175,000 calories

175,000 calories as a percentage of 7,300,000 = 0.2 percent

That's not much. In theory, the man in our example erred in matching his calories in and calories out by only 0.2 percent. Obviously, the body can strike a fine balance, and it's this balancing process, not the calories in/calories out equation, that should fascinate us. This built-in balancing process means that our bodies have the wisdom to tell us to eat when we are hungry, to select nutritious food, and to stop when we've eaten enough. Sadly, we don't always heed their advice. Imagine! Millions of people with no knowledge of nutritional science and without the means to measure or weigh themselves have achieved the amazing feat of balancing their energy without even thinking about it. Really, you can do it, too, and you can do it without counting calories, weighing and measuring yourself, scoring points, or carrying around a calorie-counting table. It's just as Arthur Frank testified in the case of Bonnie Cook: He doesn't pay any attention to what he eats; he eats only what he likes and stops when he feels satisfied. And he has maintained a stable weight for the last 20 years.

Fat Trap: The Old Energy Equation

In an effort to understand the flux of energy in the body, researchers applied the science of physics to the human body. The First Law of Thermodynamics states that energy cannot be created or destroyed, only transferred. For example, plants absorb energy from the sun and grow. Small animals eat the plants, consuming the energy they obtained from the sun. Then large animals eat the small animals, and so on, with energy transferring up the food chain.

Researchers originally thought the same principle applied to the food we eat and that what went in must come out in perfect balance. If more goes in than comes out, you gain weight. If more comes out than goes in, you lose weight. You can picture it like the figures that follow.

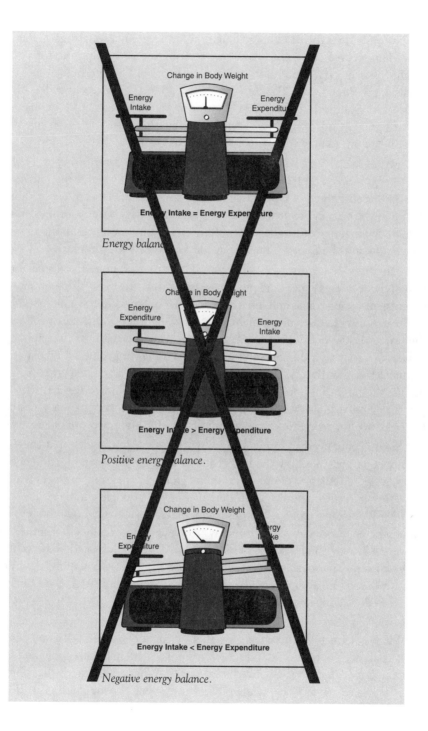

Energy balance.

Positive energy balance.

Negative energy balance.

Not only does the old Energy Equation fail to predict weight gain, but it also fails to predict weight loss. Using the old Energy Equation to forecast weight loss seemed a straightforward matter. Because 1 pound human fat equals approximately 3,500 calories, to lose 1 pound you merely needed to reduce your energy intake by 500 calories per day for a week until—voilà!— you've lost a pound.[3] Well, anybody who has ever tried to lose weight by reducing calories knows that this doesn't always work.

In the past, if somebody went to a nutritionist and described eating habits and energy intake at a level ideal for a person half their weight, the nutritionist would accuse them of lying. Medical practitioners have been taught that the Energy Equation dictates weight loss, and that's the only tool they can use to fight the metabolic disorders that often accompany overweight and obesity. So why doesn't the Energy Equation work, and what's the alternative?

Scientists are beginning to understand that there is more to our metabolism and our energy-balancing processes than meets the eye. Although many experiments using the simple Energy Equation theory seem to support it, now evidence shows that neither weight gain nor weight loss consistently follow the Energy Equation's logic.[4,5,6] The trouble is, sometimes it does. In science, somebody proposes a theory, and then a lot of different people set up experiments to test that theory. But as long as some of them do, an expert can dismiss the ones that don't as experimental "noise" or imprecise scientific practice. This explains why the old Energy Equation proponents have ignored the evidence that sometimes the metabolism defies their accepted logic.

Even experienced and up-to-date scientists cling to the idea that the Energy Equation rules how the body balances energy. For example, Steven Jonas, M.D., a professor of preventative medicine at the State University of New York and the co-author of *Just the Weight You Are: How to Be Fit and Healthy, Whatever Your Size,*[7] refuses to denounce the Energy Equation, even though he acknowledges that "in many overweight people, metabolism is not 'Standard,' to say the least."[8] Carl Foster, Ph.D., a professor at the University of Wisconsin–La Crosse, says that just because the Energy Equation "doesn't work, it doesn't mean it's invalid." However, he, too, admits that the Energy Equation doesn't adequately explain what really happens in weight loss and gain.[9]

Many scientists are now realizing that our metabolism and the way our bodies balance energy do not adhere to a simple mathematical model and are far more complex than they once had thought. What goes in and what comes out is only a fraction of the whole biological system. No one knows the full, complicated story yet, especially as it applies differently to each of the millions of individuals who want to lose weight.

When we don't understand the full story, we can nevertheless apply the "black box theory." Imagine human metabolism as an "energy black box." We don't fully understand how it functions, but we can examine what goes in and what comes out. Through trial and error, we can learn what helps or hurts the system. Sometimes we observe unexpected results. It's still mysterious. No two individuals are identical. That said, we can use the energy black box to help us develop a new way of thinking about the metabolism and how the body balances energy, to free us from the old dogma and replace it with a new approach based on how the body really does work.

The Energy Black Box

The energy black box simplifies a complex system of metabolic, emotional, and physical variables that differs from person to person. Together, these variables determine whether our metabolism is fast or slow, whether we gain or lose weight, and whether we feel highly energized or constantly fatigued. In fact, all the observations you made in "Activity 2.2: Monitor Your Metabolism" are the result of what is going on inside your energy black box. We don't yet understand all the interactions that happen inside the energy black box, but we do understand how to use the energy black box to help change our lives.

The following figure represents what goes on inside our bodies, all the mechanisms and processes of the metabolism and weight regulation. On the left side of the diagram, you see the energy we take in: what we eat. On the right side, you see the ways we use energy: what we do. Resting metabolic rate is the amount of energy you expend while lying down and doing nothing. Thermogenesis refers to the generation of heat for warmth and the energy needed to digest food.

Unlike the old model of energy balancing in the body, in which a simple pivot point sits between the energy in and the energy out, the energy black box is far more complex. Many factors affect how well the systems within the energy black box operate:

- **Emotions.** Stress releases hormones that tell the body to conserve energy. If you live a life of high stress, you may have noticed a weight gain.
- **Genetics.** A host of genetic factors make us more or less susceptible to weight gain. Although we can't do anything about these, we can design strategies for coping with them.

- **Environmental conditioning.** The way our parents taught us to eat powerfully influences our eating habits. For example, did your parents always tell you to clean your plate, whether you wanted to or not? Our habits become surprisingly ingrained: We eat what we've always eaten because we know what we like and how to cook it. One study found that out of the millions of foods available to us in our supermarkets, most of us eat the same 28 foods every week. We are creatures of habit.

- **Surrounding environment.** If you encounter a restaurant every 100 yards on your way home from work, you'll find it harder to ignore them all and go home to prepare a nutritious meal. If the television bombards you with 10 ads for tasty snack food an hour, you'll find it hard not to think about food. If the restaurant puts more food on your plate than you really want, you'll find it hard not to eat it all. Our whole culture seems intent on telling us to eat, eat, and eat some more.

- **Medications.** Many common medications interfere with metabolism and the hormonal regulation of weight. Taking birth control pills can affect weight, as can amphetamines and hundreds of other frequently prescribed drugs.

- **Recreational/lifestyle drugs.** Cigarette smoking can boost the metabolism by 10 percent and curb the appetite, but you end up losing essential nutrients. Caffeine can raise your metabolism briefly, but the low that follows often causes you to reach for a sugary snack later. Studies have shown that when you consume alcohol with a meal, you always eat more than if you drink plain water. All these self-prescribed drugs cause subtle yet important effects on your energy-balancing mechanisms.

- **Climate.** Some people burn more calories in a cooler climate or find exercise more amenable when they don't have to cope with heat and humidity. Others can't get out the door unless they feel the sun on their backs.

- **Social surroundings.** We are influenced by our friends and family. For example, how often have you asked the person you're dining with whether they're ordering an appetizer or a dessert before you commit to ordering one yourself? Generally, we fall in with our companions. If they have developed bad food habits, so will we.

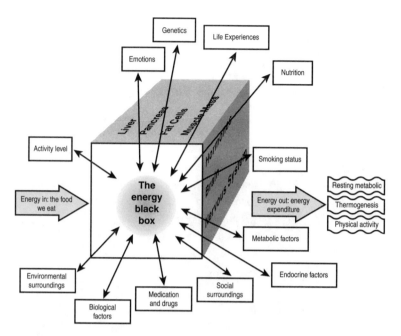

The Energy Black Box.

Influences on the Energy Black Box

The following list represents the range of factors that can affect our metabolism and our energy-balancing mechanisms.

Category	Influence
Emotions	Stress
	Anger
	Body image
	Abuse
	Loneliness
	Love, passion
	Fear
	Anxiety
Environment	Climate: hot, cold, humid, dry
	Noise and light pollution

	Availability of different types of food
	Quality of available food—nutrient-dense or nutrient-poor
	Toxicity in the environment—poisons
Genetics	Inherited body type
	Inherited metabolism type, circulation, digestive enzymes
Illnesses, medications, and drugs	Illnesses that affect energy—diabetes, cancer, heart disease, eating disorders
	Medications for other illnesses that affect energy
	Recreational drug use
	Lifestyle drug use, including coffee, cigarettes, alcohol
	Addictions to caffeine, alcohol, nicotine, sugar
	Allergies
Experiences in life	Prebirth nutritional conditioning
	Early life behavioral conditioning
	Abuse
	Knowledge of nutrition
	Skills in food preparation
	Past physical conditioning
Social surroundings	Intimate, close relationships
	Social group
	Social habits
	Work environment and demands
	Pressure to consume food and alcohol
	Cultural/religious traditions
	Recreational choices
	Family roles and commitments

Using the framework of the energy black box, weight gain is not merely a matter of eating too much or exercising too little. It also depends on what goes on inside the black box—how our bodies operate. These incompletely understood processes and feedback mechanisms can explain why some people don't lose weight even on an extremely low-calorie diet, why at a certain stage in your life you can suddenly gain weight, and why health and lifestyle affect weight regulation.

For example, stress and negative emotions can make us fat. When we feel threatened, fearful, worried, anxious, and angry, the body responds by hoarding energy. Levels of the stress hormone cortisol rise and turn off fat burning. When we remain in a constant state of "fight or flight" preparedness, our body responds by hoarding its principle means of survival: body fat.

Subtle but significant hormone imbalances also affect what our bodies do with what we eat. For example, depressed levels of thyroid hormones, at levels undetectable by blood tests, can lead to a slowing of the metabolism sufficient to cause weight gain; so can a small overproduction of the hormone melatonin. The changes in female sex hormones that accompany puberty, childbearing, and menopause can cause a huge shift in metabolism. Illness, pollution, nutritional deficiencies, certain foods, and medications can all affect the delicate balance of our metabolic hormones. A diet too dependent on simple carbohydrates, even if it does not contain excessive calories, can affect our insulin sensitivity and lead to metabolic malfunctioning.

Managing Weight with the Energy Black Box

Many people come to my seminars with concerns about weight loss. They want to know how a heart rate monitor can help them with their weight management. My stock answer? You shouldn't be trying to manage your weight; you should be trying to manage your energy black box. When you try to manage weight, based on the old Energy Equation model of weight loss/ gain, you only manipulate energy intake (calorie-controlled diets) or energy output (increasing physical activity). Most dieters have learned that this rather unsophisticated approach rarely succeeds in the long term. In contrast, when you manage your energy black box, you manipulate three factors: energy in, energy out, and, crucially, what happens inside the black box.

Eat right, exercise right, develop a properly functioning energy black box, and your body naturally finds its own healthy weight. You don't "manage your weight"; you take simple steps to ensure that the processes within the black box can run smoothly and that your body's built-in natural energy balancing processes can work naturally. Your "healthy weight" may or may not be less than you weigh now or match the so-called "ideal" weight for your height. When you base it on your energy black box, however, you can be sure that it's a weight you can sustain, that you'll have a lot of energy, and that it contributes to your all-around health.

Developing a Properly Functioning Energy Black Box

When people start to grasp the concept of the energy black box and change their approach to weight issues, something amazing happens: They get a huge energy boost. I have seen it happen hundreds of times. By managing the processes within the black box and making subtle changes in the way they eat, they shift their energy levels. You, too, can apply "energy-shifting" techniques to manage your own energy black box.

Energy Shifting

Energy shifting is not about dieting; it's about doing things differently. What things? You can do literally hundreds of things to adjust the factors affecting your energy black box, from altering your energy input and output to modifying what happens between what goes into your energy black box and what comes out. Not all strategies will work for all people. The ones that work for you will be unique to you. To find them, you must experiment: Try new things, discern what doesn't suit you, and keep tinkering until you get the results you want. You can use the observations you made in "Activity 2.2: Monitor Your Metabolism" to guide you toward making positive changes. Effective energy shifting works best if you address one mechanism or process at a time. If a change works, keep it in your bag of fitness tricks. If not, forget it and select another variable to test on yourself. Some experiments you might conduct on your unique body include the following:

Energy shifting on the energy-in side:

- Change your eating patterns. Look at your meal timing to see if you can change anything that will provide more energy when you need it and keep you from gorging on food you don't need because you got too hungry. Graze, don't feast—that is, eat many smaller meals rather than a few large ones.

- Examine your consumption of high-fat foods. High-fat foods contain a lot of calories and taste great. That makes it easy to eat too much of them. Try replacing high-fat foods with lower-fat alternatives.

- Choose nutrient-dense whole foods. Avoid foods that contain empty calories. Eat foods that give you nutrients, vitamins, and minerals.

- Reduce the sugar in your diet. Research has shown that simple carbohydrates like sugar satisfy you less, causing you to eat more of them.

- Adjust the percentages of carbohydrates, protein, and fat in your diet. Experiment and try different foods. Some people eat less if they eat the right things. Try eating more meat or less meat, or more raw food or more complex carbohydrates.
- Exercise more. Research has shown that people who exercise choose a better, more nutritious diet than people who don't exercise.

Energy shifting on the energy-output side:

- Do not restrict your calorie intake or go hungry for long stretches of time. When you do this, your body conserves energy.
- Keep your fuel tanks topped up with energy. Eat breakfast and keep your energy up throughout the day by grazing rather than feasting on big meals.
- Reduce your television and computer time.
- Increase your daily physical activity.
- Exercise for longer periods and at a higher intensity.
- Build your lean body mass through resistance training, which will increase your resting metabolic rate.

Energy shifting in the black box:

- Get adequate rest and sleep.
- Reduce stress.
- Schedule more time with those you love.
- Reduce medications, drugs, coffee, alcohol, and cigarettes.
- Improve your body image.
- Address emotional issues.
- Enhance social surroundings and loving relationships.
- Eat a diet with adequate vitamins and minerals, to ensure that you have no nutritional deficiencies.
- Try to alleviate food allergies or digestive problems by changing your diet.
- Reduce your intake of harmful fats, and increase your intake of beneficial fats.
- Reduce environmental toxins by eating organic produce, avoiding food kept in soft plastic, filtering water, eliminating charred food, and minimizing time spent in smoggy traffic or smoky atmospheres.

Universal Black Box Rules

While no two people share the same energy black boxes and must therefore find their own individual ways of manipulating their black boxes, it turns out that several fundamental principles are universal to everybody.

Universal Principle 1: Don't Restrict Calories

When you diet (restricting the number of calories you put in your body each day), you initiate a cascade of biochemical changes that will undermine your long-term weight status and metabolic health, your immediate emotional health, and your current energy levels. The body responds to dieting the same way it responds to starvation. It can't understand that you just want to slim down: That doesn't compute in its programming.

For the body, starvation sends a signal to "man the panic stations." For a start, your body turns off fat burning. Next, it raises the levels of the stress hormones, which interferes with your ability to build muscle, impedes the proper functioning of insulin, and slows your metabolism. Next, your body puts all essential repairs on hold. Your body may stop being able to absorb and process essential vitamins and minerals even if you add these to your low-calorie diet as supplements. Now a food obsession develops, in which you think about food all the time and crave unhealthful foods. When you do eat, you don't select the right quality and quantity of food. Finally your cognitive ability declines. You can't concentrate well or think clearly, and your emotions are on edge. As a result, both your mood and your relationships suffer.

Universal Principle 2: You Have a Unique Biological Makeup

Imagine that for two weeks you're caring for a Labrador Retriever and a Greyhound. Now suppose that you give exactly the same food and training to both dogs. What would happen? One of the dogs would most likely gain weight, while the other would stay the same weight. Why? The Greyhound and the Labrador have completely different metabolisms. The same applies to people. No two biological makeups—no two black boxes—are the same. The type or quantity of food, the lifestyle, and the mode of physical activity that could be right for one person might be totally wrong for another. Therefore, we must become our own physiologists, experimenting to find what works best for our unique bodies.

Universal Principle 3: Make Small Incremental Changes

Whatever metabolic, physical, and emotional changes you choose for your life, you should make them slowly and continuously. Long-term change usually depends on making small, progressive changes frequently. The Japanese have a word for it: *kaizen*, which means 1 percent change a hundred times. Sure, you might dream of overnight change, but the body resists rapid change. Take 100 steps toward 100 percent change.

Universal Principle 4: Eat a Balanced Diet

Your body cannot function well unless you eat a balanced diet. What does this look like? Well, you probably know most of the principles already:

- Eat small, frequent meals containing a balance of protein, carbohydrate, and fat. (I'll cover this in more depth when we get to Chapter 5.)
- Make the majority of your diet whole foods.
- Limit your consumption of refined carbohydrates.
- Limit harmful fats, such as saturated fats and partially hydrogenated fats.
- Eat plenty of beneficial fats, including cold-water fish, nuts, and seeds.
- Consume plenty of fresh fruit and vegetables.
- Select a wide variety of foods prepared in different ways.
- Drink plenty of water.

Everyone can follow these basic nutritional guidelines. And everyone can tailor their particular plan to their unique desires and tastes. Only you can discern your own perfect way of eating. Listen to your body. It knows what's good for it, provided that you pay close attention to it.

Activity 4.3: Taking Five Steps to Shift Your Energy

A step-by-step approach to energy shifting offers the most practical way to change the way that your energy black box operates. If you really want to get healthier, to get fitter, and to improve your energy levels, you need to shift your energy progressively until your biological makeup escalates to a new state of homeostasis.

Step 1: Analyze Your Life

With the diagram of the energy black box in mind, review your results from Activity 4.1. Try to identify any areas of your life that have gotten out of balance. Are they on the energy-getting side, inside the black box, or on the energy-taking side? What are the major influences on your life? Examine family constraints, your work environment, and your past experience. How about stress or negative emotions?

Activity 4.3. *continued*

Can you see any genetic factors that influence your life, such as overweight parents or family members with high blood pressure? Have you let your social surroundings override your natural intuitive processes? Be ruthlessly honest with yourself. You might ask a close friend to help you talk through your life and all the factors that might be affecting it right now. We make lasting changes more easily with the support of loved ones.

Wear your heart rate monitor while you are taking Step 1. It will give you valuable feedback on how you really feel about different areas of your life. Jot down your observations in your personal fitness log.

Step 2: Collect a Bag of Tricks

When you have identified problematic areas where you want to make changes, you can use any number of tools to help you find solutions. Think of these tools as your personal bag of tricks. Your own bag will include the techniques that work for your unique body and situation. Choose some energy shifting tricks from the list I've compiled, or use your own tricks that you know from experience work for you. You could even get some ideas from your friends. Whichever ideas you choose, you will want to match them to the list of major influences you identified in Step 1.

Don't just pick tools you like, such as getting a massage, or that are unrealistic, such as taking up skiing if you live in Florida. Choose tricks that suit your life and fit your biological makeup and that you can realistically implement. Can you come up with 10 tricks that might work for you? Write your list of 10 tricks using the form in Appendix F.

The bag of tricks:

1. Take a weekend class, go on a retreat, or enroll in an evening seminar at your local learning center on topics such as body image, emotional stability, ways to express love, or stress and anger management.

2. Read a book on a new fitness activity that you have always dreamed of, such as Pilates, triathlon, snowshoeing, or stretching.

3. Get a pet or borrow a friend's pet for a day.

4. Ask your friends about how they perceive your current lifestyle, and ask them for their input. Sometimes you have to ask for help.

5. Ask yourself whether your environment is suitable and what you might do to improve it.

6. Consider your wardrobe and ask yourself whether it is time to wear clothes that allow for more movement. Are the shoes you wear designed for comfort and movement?

7. Get a massage biweekly for eight weeks.

8. Look at your vacation schedule. Do you take enough time away from your everyday life? If you can't take two weeks off, how about a series of long weekend minivacations?

9. What can you do to reduce the toxicity in your environment? Can you walk when the particle count in the air is lowest? Are you drinking filtered water? Is your home free from environmental pollution?

10. Determine your basic body type: are you a Greyhound or a Labrador; a Thoroughbred or a Clydesdale? Do your activities match your body type?

11. Read the labels on what you eat and consciously purchase items that fit with your eating choices.

12. Change the foods you eat, and try different dietary regimens, such as eating six small meals a day rather than three larger ones.

13. Add more fruit and vegetables to your diet.

14. Wear a heart rate monitor while eating and drinking. Do your heart rate numbers change when you consume certain foods or drinks?

15. Ask yourself (and your medical professionals) whether you need to take the current pills and dosages that you have been prescribed.

16. Read about vitamins and mineral supplements, and begin to take those that you believe will improve your physiology.

17. Change your sleeping patterns by adding or subtracting from the number of hours you currently sleep.

18. Take something out of your diet: caffeine, nicotine, alcohol, or simple carbohydrates, for example.

19. Join a group that does fun, new activities such as dancing, going on weekend adventures, reading, or meditating.

Activity 4.3. *continued*

20. Ask a family member or friend to join you in a new activity.

21. Change the number of hours that you work on a computer or watch television.

22. Set aside time to spend with your children or a friend's children.

23. Volunteer your time and your money for a social or health cause that makes you feel that you are contributing to a better world.

24. Set an attainable fitness goal.

25. Tell someone verbally or in writing that you love them.

Here's Lorraine's bag of tricks:

- Go to the health club in the morning instead of staying in bed.

- Take more food to work from home.

- Change the main meal from dinner to lunch.

- Do not go out for restaurant dinners so often.

- Alter wine-drinking habits: one glass of wine when at the pub. Drink wine only on the weekend. Drink wine at home only when entertaining.

- Buy a new mountain bike.

- Get a heart rate monitor and do every fitness workout with it.

- Schedule several periodic fitness assessments at the health club.

- Eat more in the afternoons to get more energy for evening workouts.

- Set some physical fitness goals.

- Start weight training to improve muscle mass.

- Buy some new workout clothes so I feel better going to the club.

Step 3: Prioritize

Most of us live in a time-starved world. That's one good reason for you to set priorities, making sure you actually do accomplish the most important changes you've decided to tackle. But which ideas are the best and deserve your fullest effort? Some may need more thought and preparation than others. Some may be more effective at shifting your energy than others. To help you set your priorities, list each trick on the chart and give it a score between 1 and 5 for how effective you think it will be. A blank chart is provided for you in Appendix F. Then add a score for how easily you think you can implement it. Multiplying the two scores will give you a number that will help you assign a priority to the trick.

The Priority Game

This game makes prioritizing fun and easy. Just follow these simple directions:

Column A: List each item in your bag of tricks.

Column B: Score each trick according to its potential effectiveness: 5 for most effective in boosting energy levels, and 1 for small changes in energy levels.

Column C: Score each trick according to how easily you think you could implement it: 1 for difficult, and 5 for very easy.

Column D: Multiply Column B by Column C to determine an overall score.

Column E: Rank the results, using the highest number in Column D as the highest priority for you. Begin implementing this trick today.

When Lorraine played this game, hoping to achieve more energy, less stress, and improved fitness, she got these results:

Lorraine's Priority Game

(A) Tricks	(B) Effectiveness	(C) Difficulty	(D) Score	(E) Ranking
Energy tricks	Potential effectiveness (1 = not very; 5 = very effective	Implemen- tation (1 = hard; 5 = easy)	Score (multiply column 1 and 2)	Rank (highest number = highest priority)
Go to the health club in the morning instead of staying in bed.	5	2	10	8
Take more food to work from home.	4	4	16	3
Change the main meal from dinner to lunch.	3	3	9	10

Activity 4.3. *continued*

(A) Tricks	(B) Effectiveness	(C) Difficulty	(D) Score	(E) Ranking
Energy tricks	Potential effectiveness (1 = not very; 5 = very effective	Implemen- tation (1 = hard; 5 = easy)	Score (multiply column 1 and 2)	Rank (highest number = highest priority)
Do not go out for restaurant dinners so often.	4	3	12	6
Alter wine-drinking habits: one glass of wine when at the pub. Drink wine only on the weekend. Drink wine at home only when entertaining.	3	5	15	4
Buy a new mountain bike	4	2	8	11
Get a heart rate monitor and do every fitness workout with it.	5	5	25	1
Schedule several peri- odic fitness assessments at the health club.	3	3	9	10
Eat more in the after- noons to get more energy for evening workouts.	4	5	20	2
Set some physical fitness goals.	5	3	15	4
Start weight training to improve muscle mass.	4	3	12	6
Buy some new workout clothes so I feel better going to the club.	2	5	10	8

Lorraine's final list of priorities for her chosen energy-shifting activities are given next. Write yours in the list provided in Appendix F.

Lorraine's Final List of Prioritized Energy-Shifting Activities

Priority No.	Activity
1	Got a heart rate monitor and did every fitness workout with one.
2	Ate more in the afternoons so had energy to work out in the evenings.
3	Decided to take more food to work from home.
4	Set some physical fitness goals.
5	Set up deals about drinking wine:
	Only one glass of wine when at the pub.
	Drink wine only on the weekend.
	Drink wine at home only if guests are visiting.
6	Started weight training to improve muscle mass.
7	Did not go out for restaurant dinners so much.
8	Bought some new workout clothes so I felt better going to the club to work out.
9	Started to go to the health club in the morning instead of staying in bed.
10	Scheduled several periodic fitness assessments at the health club.
11	Changed the main meal from dinner to lunch.
12	Decided to buy a new mountain bike.

Step 4: Implement Your Priorities One Step at a Time

Now it's time to put your energy-shifting tricks into practice and see what happens. Remember that small steps will get you where you want to go. Practice "kaizen." One hundred small steps will add up to one giant step.

For example, you might decide to take a small step by choosing to replace a midafternoon candy snack with a midafternoon fruit snack. That results in energy shifting. Try it to see what happens. Don't think of this energy-shifting activity as

---

Activity 4.3. *continued*

denial of candy; it isn't denial. In fact, don't do anything you feel is denial. Do only things you think will improve your health.

Step 5: Experiment with Your Biological Makeup

Get feedback from your emotional, physical, and metabolic heart. Observe the effect of energy-taking changes on your energy giving. Play with your bag of tricks and your black box. Use the observations you made on your metabolism in "Activity 2.2: Monitor Your Metabolism" to help guide you toward a metabolism that works better for you. You'll certainly accomplish more if you're having fun gaining more knowledge about your biological makeup.

Week 3 Summary

By the end of this week, you should be making some changes with respect to your own energy levels, your unique energy black box, and your strategies for encouraging your physiology and biochemistry to work more effectively for you. You've learned something about how the body balances its energy, and you should have gained a new outlook on your fatness, viewing it in the context of influences on your black box and not simply as a personal failure that sparks guilt. You've got your work cut out for you implementing your bag of tricks. In the next chapter, I'll introduce you to ways you can use your new-found levels of energy for specific types of training. For now, keep moving and shift your energy!

CHAPTER 5

Week 4: Metabolic Fitness
Maximizing Vitality, Minimizing Disease

The focus of this chapter is metabolic fitness, the next physical and emotional fitness. In your first week, you started to move; in your second week, you completed your first training workouts; and during week 3, you learned about energy shifting. Now we want to explore how training can give you key metabolic benefits. Those benefits include reducing a tendency toward becoming insulin-resistant and eventually developing type II diabetes, lowering blood pressure, improving your blood lipid profile, and reducing your cholesterol. All these lower your risk of developing cardiovascular heart disease and diabetes. We'll also discuss the significance of sugar and fat in our diet. Finally, we'll do some metabolic training. It's easy, it's fun, and it's loaded with benefits.

Fitness Fights Metabolic Disease: Doreen's Story

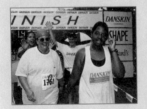

Doreen, a 36-year-old living in Chicago, had never really worried about her fitness. With obese parents and 15 obese brothers and sisters, she had never had a fitness role model, either. Type II diabetes ran in the family, so it was not a big surprise when Doreen, too, was diagnosed with the disease. One hundred fifty pounds overweight, and feeling hopeless about dealing with the problem because of her family's history of diabetes, Doreen was tempted to sit back and accept this new blight on her life. She'd just play the hand that fate had dealt her.

Then her sister-in-law suggested that she join in a training group called Team Dream, composed mainly of African American women training for a sprint distance triathlon, a race in which competitors swim 500 m, bike 20 km, and run 5 km. Every woman on the team was living an adventure of discovering the athlete inside. At first Doreen thought, "No, I can't swim. I'll drown." When her sister-in-law persisted, Doreen remained skeptical. "No way," she told her sister-in-law. "Why would I do that? I would be sure to finish last, and what would be the point of that?" Because of her size, Doreen found it challenging just to do day-to-day tasks. How could she possibly take part in a sporting event requiring consecutive swimming, biking, and running? When her sister-in-law would not take "no" for an answer, Doreen decided to attend one workout. After seeing the support and camaraderie among a group of women all striving to reach the same goal—some of them even larger and fatter than she—and after accepting the challenge of doing something about her body for the first time, she changed her mind and joined Team Dream.

Doreen started, ever so slowly, to train. Her team mates, 150 other women, cheered her every step of the way. Ninety days later, she found herself standing on the starting line of her first triathlon, as the first person in her family to take part in an athletic event. In the months before she reached the starting line, Doreen had reduced her symptoms of diabetes and had shed 90 pounds from her frame. She still had big fenders, but she had discovered and developed a big engine under her hood.

As Doreen crossed the finish line of her first triathlon, she was overcome by emotions of joy, pride, surprise, sadness, and regret, hope for the future, and just pure elation as her fellow team members and a crowd of more than 5,000 people screamed encouragement, cheered, and applauded her achievement. One of the people standing at the finish line was Doreen's 11-year-old son, an obese and unathletic kid facing a life of continued fatness, inactivity, and heightened risk of diabetes. Now he was crying, too, at his mom's incredible accomplishment and wondering if he could match it one day.

Doreen had thought she was too fat to get fit. She had struggled with weight issues all her life but had remained sedentary, falling victim at a young age to diabetes. With nothing to lose, Doreen gave fitness a chance and, wow, did it work wonders in her life! Her metabolic fitness improved, her diabetic symptoms declined, she lost a lot of weight, she became more physically capable in her everyday life, she gained self-assurance from knowing she could train for and achieve her goal. She had also made an incredible emotional impact on her family, especially her son.

Doreen is a perfect example of the fact that you can never be too fat to improve your fitness and that you don't have to be thin to take up a fitness program. She demonstrated what anyone with extra fat can accomplish, and she experienced some of the many benefits that can change our lives when we live a more active life. You are not too fat to get fit. And there is no better time than right now to implement your Fit *and* Fat Personal Activity Program and gain the huge rewards of greater metabolic, emotional, and physical health.

Understanding Metabolic Fitness

Your metabolism is the sum of all the body's biochemical processes that affect energy. When you achieve metabolic fitness, all your biochemical processes work well and you enjoy good health and great energy. The processes begin with the enzymes in your digestive tract that help digest your food. It's processes also include the way nutrients are transferred into the blood, how the cells pick up and use nutrients, and how the body stores nutrients, how the body uses nutrients from storage, and the signals it gives you to take on more nutrients, i.e., your appetite. Because everybody's metabolism is unique, the words *normal* or *average* do not apply. You'll recall that you monitored your metabolism in Chapter 2. Take a few moments now to review what you learned about your unique metabolism. Only you can get to know your metabolism and make it work to your advantage.

At a high level of metabolic fitness, your metabolism maximizes your vitality and minimizes your risk of disease; you have the energy to do what you need to do and want to do with vitality and enthusiasm. Thus, you can measure metabolic fitness in terms of energy level. At one end of the scale, a super metabolism gives you lots of energy, great health, and the ability to efficiently burn the food you eat. Halfway down the scale, your metabolism functions less well than it should, making you feel sluggish and causing you to gain weight. Further down the scale, your body chemistry becomes so deficient or imbalanced that the body grows susceptible to hormonal disorders such as hypothyroidism (depressed activity of the thyroid gland), progesterone/estrogen imbalances, abnormal blood sugar, and digestive problems such as candidiasis (infection in the gut), enzyme deficiencies, or food intolerance. Left untreated, a poorly functioning metabolism can contribute to the development of serious metabolic diseases such as type II diabetes and cardiovascular heart disease. For most individuals, the conditions that occur when your metabolism functions poorly conspire toward weight gain.

Measuring Your Metabolic Fitness

Of course, we can measure levels of metabolic fitness more scientifically. It's important to do so because, as Martin Budd warns in his book *Why Can't I Lose Weight?* health problems that coincide with weight gain might be symptoms of a depressed metabolism. Many people can solve mild problems themselves with certain lifestyle changes. More serious problems require medical care. Pause for a couple minutes and think about any symptoms you might display. If you say "yes" to any of them, seek medical help. Doctors may be able to identify and treat the underlying causes and help get you back on the road to metabolic fitness.

Identifying Metabolic Problems

Symptoms	Possible Causes
Weight gain and fatigue	Hypothyroidism, low blood sugar, candidiasis (inflammation of the digestive tract)
Weight gain with a monthly pattern	Sex hormone imbalance
Weight gain following antibiotics	Enzyme deficiency, leaky gut, or food intolerance
Weight gain and indigestion	Candidiasis, hypothyroidism, enzyme deficiency, or food intolerance

Good metabolic health can be measured using these three parameters of your health:

- Glucose tolerance and insulin sensitivity
- Blood pressure
- Blood lipids

Each of these metabolic health factors is also a key risk factor for diabetes and heart disease, two of the biggest killers in our society.

Look at the facts. Cardiovascular disease is the leading cause of death in the United States, accounting for 45 percent of all deaths in 1994. Although diabetes is only the nation's seventh leading cause of death, contributing to 187,800 deaths in 1995, medical professionals consider it the second biggest health risk factor because it increases the risk of cardiovascular disease by up to three times. Eighty percent of people with diabetes die of cardiovascular disease.[1] In addition, diabetes is the industrialized world's leading cause of blindness, kidney disease, and nontraumatic limb amputations.[2] Blood pressure, while not strictly a metabolic parameter, is also a risk factor for heart disease and diabetes.

Appreciating the Importance of Insulin Sensitivity

Despite all the complexities of human metabolism, the crux of metabolic fitness boils down to one word: *insulin*. The cornerstone of our metabolism, insulin enables our bodies to utilize the food we eat, to build muscle, to store fat, and to regulate blood sugar levels in the form of glucose. The brain needs a constant supply of glucose in order to function. Insulin sustains life. However, too much insulin can cause a multitude of problems.

The normal action of insulin helps manage your blood sugar level. For instance, when you eat a meal containing carbohydrates, the body quickly digests and absorbs glucose into the blood stream. The glucose circulates to the cells of the body. As glucose rises, the pancreas releases insulin into the blood. The insulin tells the cells to take glucose out of the blood. When the cells are healthy and react appropriately to the insulin, they are termed insulin-sensitive. When the body calls for glucose, it releases another hormone, glucagon, which tells the liver it can let some of the glucose into the blood again.

Sometimes, however, this whole process goes haywire: The cells become insulin-resistant. This often occurs when we consume too many foods containing simple sugars. Eat a lot of sugar, and the blood gets a huge rush of glucose from digestion, resulting in a high level of glucose in the blood. This imperils the body because now the pancreas must react immediately and flood the cells with insulin to get the glucose levels back under control. If blood glucose levels continue to be too high, the pancreas responds by pumping out more and more insulin. At first, this strategy works. The cells suck up the glucose, and blood sugar levels return to normal. However, when this happens repeatedly, the cells start to ignore this constant bombardment of insulin. The pancreas produces ever higher amounts of insulin, but to no avail. Now you're insulin-resistant. Between 60 and 75 million Americans are insulin-resistant, most without even realizing it. Eventually, the pancreas simply gets exhausted from the extra workload of frequently manufacturing and pumping out a huge quantity of insulin. The organ gets worn out and eventually stops making enough insulin. This signals the onset of type II diabetes. But there's some good news: The earlier insulin resistance is detected, the better our chances are of correcting the situation.

Raised glucose and insulin levels pose a serious health threat. Excess insulin raises blood pressure, lowers the beneficial fats in the blood, and increases the harmful fats in the blood. Uncontrolled high levels of insulin also make the blood more susceptible to clotting. All this raises the risk of life-threatening cardiovascular disease. Some scientists have even linked insulin levels to cancer[3]. This whole cluster of risk factors plays such a major role in the risk of heart disease that scientists have given them their own name: Syndrome X. People with Syndrome X are at the highest risk of developing heart disease[4].

Full-fledged diabetes affects about 12 million Americans[5] and 22.5 million Europeans (Henderson, Mark. "Threat of Diabetes Seriously Underrated, Say Experts." *The Times Newspaper,* 4 June 2002, 4). Of course, genetics determine to some degree whether or not you might develop type II diabetes. For those who develop the disease, about 50 percent is attributable to your genes and about 50 percent attributable to your lifestyle[6]. Changing your lifestyle, which includes what you eat, your level of physical activity, and your smoking or stress behaviors, can help you prevent diabetes.

That's good news. But there's more bad news. People with high levels of insulin tend to gain weight. Why? Insulin promotes fat storage. High insulin levels force your body into constant "food storage" mode, where you can gain weight even if you don't eat very many calories or very much food. Over the same number of years that it takes to develop diabetes, many people gain a lot of weight. This explains why a lot of people who develop diabetes are fat and why some researchers mistakenly say that obesity *causes* diabetes. Fat is a *symptom* of the underlying metabolic disorder, not the *cause* of it. And because fat gain does not cause diabetes, fat loss does not counteract insulin resistance.

How about some more good news? Fitness training can effectively normalize the insulin sensitivity of your tissues. Increased physical activity, not weight loss, is the best prescription for preventing diabetes, provided that you catch it early enough.

Getting Concerned About Fat in the Blood

You have probably heard that the amount of fat in your blood reflects how healthy you are inside. You might even believe that all fats are bad. Amazingly, despite our obsession with fat-free foods, fat-loss programs, and fat-burning workouts, every year we swallow three times our own body weight in fat[7].

Fats have gotten a bad name because a disease called arteriosclerosis, commonly known as hardening of the arteries, results in fatal heart attacks and strokes. To understand how arteriosclerosis develops, imagine that bits of cholesterol and other fats swirling around inside the arteries get stuck to the arterial walls and create fatty deposits called plaque. Over time, this plaque narrows the arteries and sometimes breaks off into the bloodstream. Whenever we need extra blood flow to do something like shovel snow or climb a few flights of stairs, the now narrow arteries just can't accommodate the extra flow. The heart tries as hard as it can to give us what we need until we experience chest pain, called angina, a sign of coronary artery disease. If the fat deposit plaque grows large enough, it eventually closes off an affected blood vessel, preventing blood from reaching a specific tissue; eventually, the tissue can die. In the case of the heart, a heart attack occurs; if in the brain, a stroke occurs. In addition, if some plaque breaks away, a stroke or heart attack can occur, causing the formation of a clot that can become lodged in the brain (stroke) or heart (heart attack).

Latest Research: The New View of Arteriosclerosis, Hardening of the Arteries

For years, scientists thought that degenerative arteriosclerosis develops like pipes getting clogged with plaque buildup. However, a recent article in the *Scientific American*[8] explains that this metaphor is now rather dated. It turns out that few plaque deposits get so big that they drastically restrict blood flow. Instead, most heart attacks result from a sudden rupture of plaque into the blood stream. The free-floating plaque triggers the development of a blood clot, called a thrombus. The blood clot itself, not the plaque on the artery's walls, blocks the blood flow.

This chain of events that can lead to a heart attack or stroke starts with low-density lipoproteins (LDL). LDL is a blood protein that carries cholesterol. When the blood contains excess LDL particles, they accumulate on the walls of blood vessels. There the LDLs undergo oxidation and glycation (binding with sugars), which you might think of as butter spoiling. The cell walls hate this and call for reinforcements from the body's immune system. From here on, all hell breaks loose.

The immune system cells try their normal process of isolation and attack, but their effort only inflames the area. Inflammation itself is not bad under normal circumstances. The immune system uses it as a natural step of healing a cut or wound. As the attempt to heal progresses, a concentration of lipids builds up inside the walls of the arteries. It's a bit like having pimples on the artery walls. The spots become concentrated cores of lipids, gummed-on LDLs, and blood-clotting chemicals. Eventually, these fatty "spots" of LDLs can rupture. Then the blood-clotting chemical escapes into the blood, and a blood clot or thrombus can form. This process explains why heart attacks can strike without warning. It also explains why certain therapies meant to avert heart attacks frequently fail.

Activity 5.1: Checking Up on Your Metabolic Fitness

In Chapter 2, Activity 2.2 asked you to monitor your metabolism for one week and write down all your observations. Now review the notes you made in the context of what you just learned about metabolic health. Rank yourself on the Metabolic Fitness Continuum chart (on a scale of 1 to 10—1 equals excellent, 10 equals terrible). Base your answers on the definition of metabolic fitness as having the reserve energy to do what you need to do and want to do with vitality and enthusiasm.

Metabolic Fitness Continuum

Question:	1	2	3	4	5	6	7	8	9	10

How healthy is your metabolism now?

How healthy do you want it to be in the future?

Playing by the Numbers and Understanding Your Results

As you've no doubt concluded by now, I love using numbers to capture information. The three key metabolic fitness parameters lend themselves so nicely to numbers: blood pressure, blood lipid levels, and insulin sensitivity. If you have not visited a doctor recently to obtain these numbers, I strongly urge you to do so soon. Blood pressure is the easiest parameter to quantify, but for accuracy's sake, make sure it's done with a manually inflating arm cuff, not an electronic device. You can take your own, but the electronic blood pressure cuffs you can buy at the drug store sometimes give inaccurate readings. If you have larger arms, make sure the arm cuff fits you properly; you may need a larger size. Because your readings can fluctuate from day to day, take multiple readings and average them. If you feel at all nervous in the doctor's office, you can also register a higher number due to "white coat syndrome."

For blood lipids, you will need a simple blood test, the results of which will take some days to come back from the laboratory. Be sure to say that you want to know your levels of each of the following:

- Triglycerides
- Total cholesterol
- LDL (low-density lipoprotein)
- HDL (high-density lipoprotein)

At least one quarter of the adults in the United States might be insulin-resistant without even realizing it. If you have been leading a sedentary life and eating a diet high in fat and simple sugar and low in fiber for many years, you run a higher risk of being insulin-resistant. A blood test taken after an overnight fast can reveal whether your levels of glucose and insulin fall within the normal range. High levels of either could indicate insulin resistance.

Blood Pressure

Your blood pressure consists of two important numbers. Both measure the pressure of blood flow in your arteries. The first number, the higher one, is the systolic pressure, the pressure of blood in your arteries when the heart contracts and propels freshly oxygenated blood through the arteries. You don't want a higher than normal systolic pressure because that shows that the heart must work very hard to push blood through the arteries. The second number is the diastolic pressure, the pressure in the arteries when the heart pauses between beats to allow time for the heart chambers to fill up with blood again. You want a normal number here because the heart must fully relax before it can efficiently contract again.

Classification of High Blood Pressure

	Systolic (mm Hg)	Diastolic (mm Hg)
Optimal	120 or less	80 or less
Normal	129 or less	84 or less
High normal	130 to 139	85 to 89
High blood pressure (also termed hypertension)	140 or more	90 or more

Blood Lipids

Your blood lipid results are usually presented as milligrams of each type of blood lipid per deciliter, or 100 milliliters, of blood (mg/dL). Lipids are not soluble in water, and to travel in the blood they must be joined to proteins. Together these new structures are called lipoproteins.

The two most important types of lipoproteins are low-density (LDL) and high-density (HDL) lipoproteins. They both carry cholesterol, which is a hard, waxy substance. Neither is inherently bad when doing its normal job. LDLs normally truck cholesterol from the liver and intestines to various tissues, which use it to repair membranes or produce steroids. LDLs have been nick-named "bad cholesterol" because an overabundance harms arterial health. The high-density ones (HDL) haul cholesterol to the liver for excretion or recycling, thus earning the label "good cholesterol." You want an abundance of these.

Other lipoproteins, the ones that carry triglycerides rather than cholesterol, are the intermediate-density lipoproteins (IDL), the very low-density lipo-proteins (VLDL), and the chylomicrons. When you get a number for total cho-lesterol, the figures include both the cholesterol carrying lipoproteins and the triglyceride lipoproteins.

Rely on your doctor or health professional to evaluate and interpret your cholesterol levels, asking any questions about your numbers and the best way to reduce your individual risk of heart disease. However, the guidelines in the following table generally apply.

Interpreting Blood Lipid Numbers

Triglycerides

Less than 150 mg/dL	Normal
150 to 199 mg/dL	Borderline
200 to 499 mg/dL	High
More than 500 mg/dL	Very high

Total Cholesterol

200 mg/dL or less	Desirable
Between 200 and 239 mg/dL	Borderline high
240 mg/dL or more	Too high

HDL

Less than 40 mg/dL	Too low
More than 40 mg/dL	Beneficial, especially if above 60 mg/dL

LDL

Less than 100 mg/dL	Desirable
100 to 129 mg/dL	Near optimal/above optimal
130 to 159 mg/dL	Borderline high
160 to 189 mg/dL	High
190 mg/dL and above	Very high

If you already have heart disease, your LDL levels should be 100 mg/dL or less.

Cholesterol Ratio

Sometimes a doctor will give you a cholesterol ratio, which represents your total cholesterol number divided by the HDL number. Ideally, this ratio should be below 5 but higher than 1 (3.5 to 1 is optimal). This calculation compares the proportion of good cholesterol HDL to bad cholesterol, LDL, and triglycerides. It provides an important indicator of your risk of contracting cardiovascular disease.

Glucose Tolerance and Insulin Sensitivity

If initial tests reveal high levels of glucose and insulin, you should take a follow-up test, called a glucose tolerance test. It requires you to drink a solution containing 75 grams of glucose (about the same amount of simple sugars as in two cans of nondiet soda) and then submit to periodic blood tests over the next three hours. If you are insulin-resistant, your blood glucose levels will register much higher than normal during those three hours as your body tries to bring down the glucose levels in your blood.

For an individual with normal glucose tolerance, blood glucose will rise no higher than 140 mg/dL after a meal and then drop back down to normal, about 90 mg/dL, within 2 hours. For a person with glucose intolerance, blood sugar might rise as high as 160 mg/dL after a meal and take 30 minutes longer than normal to return to the level before the meal. Such a condition isn't yet type II diabetes, but it does deliver a big warning, telling you to change your lifestyle today or face the dire consequences tomorrow.

Moving for Metabolic Health

To have metabolic health, you need two elements: good nutrition and an active lifestyle. You learned about the eating side of metabolic health and fitness in Chapter 3, getting in touch with your internal appetite mechanisms and trying out your own bag of energy-shifting tricks that can put you on the right track to supplying your unique body with what it needs. The other component, movement or physical activity, is equally important. People with poor metabolic health have usually lost touch with the physical activity the body needs to keep metabolically, physically, and emotionally healthy. We don't all need to be trained to run a marathon, but we all need a basic level of daily physical activity to have a healthy metabolism. Moving is a basic human need.

Fitness training bestows huge benefits in terms of your metabolic health. It helps prevent the onset of insulin resistance and can reverse the progress of type II diabetes, even curing it completely. It lowers blood pressure and significantly improves blood lipid profiles.

Regular exercise helps control excess insulin because, during exercise, the muscles need glucose but don't need insulin to tell them to take it up; and hence blood glucose levels are reduced without the need for insulin. Therefore, during exercise, the pancreas doesn't need to produce so much insulin. A single exercise session can increase insulin sensitivity in the liver and muscles for up to 16 hours,[9] and prolonged exercise produces a decline in both glucose and insulin levels. In one study of people who trained vigorously, the muscles sucked up glucose at twice the rate as before for up to 10 days after the exercise.[10] Furthermore, the carrier proteins (also called insulin receptors) that help get glucose into the cells increase in number when we exercise.

That's not all. Fitness training promotes increased blood flow. It also increases the enzymes we need for burning fuel inside our cells. In another study, individuals who were already insulin-resistant but who exercised had a 30 percent less chance of developing type II diabetes compared to those who didn't. If you are a borderline type II diabetic, that means exercise can probably help you both control your insulin levels and prevent diabetes. Results from a host of other studies have been pouring in. The following are some of them:

- Researchers followed 577 individuals with insulin resistance for 6 years and found a 46 percent reduction in the risk of developing diabetes for those who exercised.
- Dietary changes and 150 minutes a week of moderate exercise reduced the risk of developing type II diabetes by 58 percent.[11]
- The response to a single session of exercise improved the action of insulin[12,13] and the lipid profile for as long as 48 to 72 hours.[14]

Fitness training offers the most effective way to improve your blood chemistry and your blood lipid profile. In particular, exercise raises the levels of good cholesterol (HDLs). Because one of the key indicators of metabolic fitness is the ratio between good cholesterol (HDL) and bad cholesterol (LDL), any rise in HDL improves this ratio. Consider some of the evidence:

- In a 1999 review of the benefits of exercise, eight different research studies found that exercise results in an improved blood lipid profile.[15]

- Another study demonstrated that exercise can have just as much of an effect on a person's lipid profile as a very low-calorie diet.[16]

- Low-intensity endurance-type training directly improves levels of blood lipids.[17]

- A recent study of 111 men and women found that those who exercised improved their blood lipid profiles, even though they lost minimal weight.[18]

Exercise training that gets you fit also improves blood pressure. Good evidence proves that exercise alone, regardless of any attendant weight loss, reduces blood pressure.[19] People without high blood pressure can expect a drop of about 3 mm Hg, and people with high blood pressure can expect a drop of up to 13 mm Hg/8 mm Hg in systolic and diastolic blood pressure, respectively. Very significantly, this effect appears to occur independently of weight loss.[20]

One further benefit of fitness training on your total metabolism is changes in your ability to metabolize fat. We'll talk more about this in Chapter 7, which deals with fat burning, but for now you just need to know that fitness training changes how you burn fat and carbohydrates. For example, metabolically fit people burn more fat when at rest and when they exercise than unfit people.

Designing Your Personal Metabolic Training Program

Exercise enhances metabolic fitness, but not all exercise brings the same benefits. Some types of exercise do more than others, and some can actually harm your metabolic health. In general, prolonged low-intensity exercise up to about 75 percent of your maximum heart rate works best. This means that training in heart zones 1, 2, and 3 will most benefit your metabolic fitness. Different things happen metabolically in the different zones.

Zone 1: Healthy Heart Zone

You enter Zone 1 when you take your heart rate above 50 percent of your maximum heart rate. A lot of metabolic magic happens within Zone 1, the Healthy Heart Zone. Many fitness experts dismiss the Healthy Heart Zone as too low of an intensity for any real physical fitness benefits. But now that we better understand human metabolism, we find strong, tangible benefits in Zone 1. The more you need the benefits of Zone 1, the more you will get from exercising in it. For people who have led sedentary lives, exercising at this intensity can be challenging, whereas trained athletes may find it too easy. Untrained athletes can realize improvements in their cardiovascular output, and trained athletes can boost their fat-burning mechanism, recovery capacity, skills, and coordination. In Zone 1, you can also have a lot of fun because you can talk while you walk, practice aspects of your sport that you don't normally do, try a new skill, mentor a less experienced athlete, and enjoy the companionship of your friends without realizing you're really exercising. The physiological changes that happen in Zone 1 include the following:

- The immune system is stimulated.
- The heart works harder and becomes stronger and more efficient.
- The muscles take up glucose from the bloodstream without needing so much insulin, reducing the need for the pancreas to produce the hormone.
- Stress is reduced, so there's less of the harmful stress hormones that encourage the body to store fat.
- Circulation improves, for more efficient transport of oxygen and nutrients to the body's tissues, and more efficient removal of waste products.
- The muscle cells take up fat more readily from the bloodstream.
- The fat deposits more readily release fat into the bloodstream for the muscles to use.
- The liver produces less "bad" cholesterol and more "good" cholesterol.
- Mood and feelings of well-being are enhanced.

Zone 2: Temperate Zone

The more challenging Zone 2 starts at 60 percent of your maximum heart rate. Though it requires more effort than the Healthy Heart Zone, it is the zone in which you can maintain exercise for a sustained period of time. Here you burn a high proportion of calories from fat, maybe up to 85 percent of the total calories burned. In the Temperate Zone, you stimulate the immune system, relieve stress, and improve the strength and efficiency of the heart muscle. The muscles become hungrier fat burners and develop more mitochondria, the parts of the cells that release energy. The capillaries to your muscles expand, carrying blood to your muscles more efficiently.

Now you are improving the way your body burns fat and mobilizes it from fat stores to muscles. Even after exercising, there is an increase in fat burning. The liver continues to increase its efficiency and the type of cholesterol it gives out. The body also reduces its requirement for insulin. Regardless of their current level of fitness or fatness, everyone experiences cardiovascular benefits while working out in the Temperate Zone. Depending on your level of fitness, you're likely to feel an emotional high from training in Zone 2.

Zone 3: Aerobic Zone

At some point in Zone 3, depending on your own physiology and current level of conditioning, the benefits start to transition from metabolic fitness to physical fitness. Here you get your heart rate up to 70 to 80 percent of your maximum. You're still burning a high proportion of calories from fat, and you're still gaining benefits in terms of fat burning, but your body will also begin to prefer glucose as a fuel. In Zone 3, the intensity of exercise produces large improvements in physical fitness and cardiovascular function. The biggest benefit of Zone 3 training is gaining the ability to exercise harder and longer at the same heart rate.

Lorraine was surprised by the benefits of training in the metabolic zones when she was preparing for her first marathon.

The Magic of Metabolic Training: Lorraine's Story

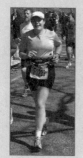

For 2002, I set for myself the goal of the Hamburg Marathon. I wasn't born a runner. I don't have the body type or the genetics. I had not run a step since childhood. Now, at age 30, I was so elated that I had finished my first running race, a 4 km road run, that soon I was doing longer distances. I set a challenge for myself of running the Marathon. I had nine months to prepare and I was determined.

I donned my heart rate monitor, set my zones, developed a plan, and worked the plan. I thought I had done everything right. I got a training partner, went to a training class, hired a coach, had my running biomechanics analyzed, bought two new pairs of running shoes, kept a log, joined a support team, let others know about my goal, and made marathon training my number-one priority. I even splurged. I bought a fancy new computer-downloadable heart rate monitor with PC Coach software to help me analyze the data.

It got to just five weeks away from the big day. I started to feel a whole series of nagging aches and pains after training. I wondered if it was my wise body telling me that I was overtraining and risking injury. I wasn't injured yet; it was just that everything hurt: The muscles in my legs continually ached, my feet and ankles were sore, and I felt drained of emotional and physical energy. Yes, my training load, my heart zones training points, had been high over the previous weeks, so I began to wonder if I should reduce my running load. But I decided to stick with my program because I thought that my body was just reacting to my training beyond what I had ever done before.

I asked a heart zones coach to look at my log book, where I had been keeping track of how much time I was spending in the different heart zones. The first thing he noticed was how much time I was spending in Zone 3 and above, and he asked me why. I answered, "I have to get faster for the marathon; I don't want to be last. There's a cutoff of 5 hours and 30 minutes, and I want to run under 5 hours, so I'm working in high zones to go faster." He pointed out to me that I hadn't been doing enough training in the lower heart zones. I hadn't been doing enough metabolic training. He was right. In my determination to get faster, and with the marathon looming closer and closer, I had lost sight of the need to incorporate metabolic training into my training schedule.

After examining the soreness in my legs, my coach gave me his final edict: "I think you've got two options if you want to do the race. Either you rest completely for a week, or you train with a heart rate below the ceiling of Zone 2 for a week." When I objected, saying I needed to get faster, not slower, he stopped me short. "No," he said, "you need to recover, not train, at the moment. If you try to train for speed now, you will get injured and will not be able to finish the race."

I decided to take his advice. I completed all of my running mileage that week below the ceiling of Zone 2, which for me is 133 bpm. It worked wonders. As the week went by, my soreness left me, my energy returned, and I recovered.

When the day came for my marathon, I warmed up at the starting line uninjured. I had reached my goal by training more in the lower heart zones. I felt like a champion when I crossed the finish line in 4 hours, 53 minutes. I, Lorraine, had succeeded using the Fit *and* Fat program. I broke five hours. I had become a marathoner. I proved that a fit and fat woman can do anything if she puts her mind to it.

Introducing Metabolic Fitness Training

Staying on a metabolic fitness-training program requires motivation, the emotional energy that turns thought into action. And nothing should motivate you more than remembering why you fitness train and what benefits you'll gain: a longer, healthier, happier life. Metabolic fitness comes from working out in heart zones 1 to 3. Follow the guidelines below when you develop your Fit *and* Fat Personal Activity Program to ensure you give yourself the opportunity to develop your optimum metabolic fitness.

- Build up your training gradually until you can sustain your heart rate within the metabolic training zones for longer periods of time. The longer the workouts in your metabolic zones are, the more you benefit from the time spent there.
- Do metabolic training at least twice per week.
- Focus on other benefits besides fitness, such as socializing, learning a new skill, training at a friend's level, and having fun.
- Engage in activities that use large muscle groups, such as walking, running, cross-country skiing, rowing, hill walking, cycling, swimming, or stepping. Whenever you rely on a large proportion of your muscle mass, you tire less easily, can keep going longer, and get more metabolic benefits from your workout.

Try the following metabolic fitness workout twice this week:

Activity 5.2: Midpoint Cha Cha Cha

Put fun into your metabolic fitness training by doing a little dancing. Put on your favorite dance music—reggae, salsa, or heavy metal. Move your feet and body until you get your heart rate to the midpoints of Zone 1, then Zone 2, then Zone 3.

Write down the midpoint for each of your three metabolic heart zones using the heart zones chart in Chapter 3 or by multiplying your maximum heart rate by the midpoint percentages.

Midpoint Zone 1: 55 percent of your maximum heart rate _____ bpm

Midpoint Zone 2: 65 percent of your maximum heart rate _____ bpm

Midpoint Zone 3: 75 percent of your maximum heart rate _____ bpm

---

Activity 5.2. *continued*

You will work out for 30 to 45 minutes, depending on your current level of fitness. The fitter you are, the longer you can sustain and enjoy your workout.

Start with a good warm-up of at least five minutes up to the midpoint of Zone 2. Dance one minute at the midpoint of Zone 1, two minutes at the midpoint of Zone 2, and three minutes at the midpoint of Zone 3. Then quickly recover back down to the midpoint of Zone 1, and begin dancing again with the same sequence: one minute at the midpoint of Zone 1, two minutes at the midpoint of Zone 2, and three minutes at the midpoint of Zone 3. Do as many repetitions as you can in 30 to 45 minutes. End your workout by gradually bringing your heart rate down to the floor of Zone 1.

If you were to draw a plot of your heart rate over your workout, it should look like that in the following figure.

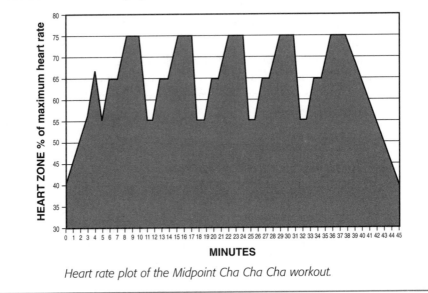

Heart rate plot of the Midpoint Cha Cha Cha workout.

Eating for Metabolic Health

What, when, how, and how much we eat can dramatically affect our metabolic fitness. That doesn't mean that we must control, count, or worry about calories or go on one of the heavily promoted weight-loss diets to realize metabolic benefits. It does mean that we should abandon ways of eating that can harm our metabolism and adopt ways of eating that can enhance it. By making simple and straightforward adjustments to our eating habits, we can magnify the benefits of metabolic fitness training.

In terms of what you eat, you should focus on two major items: dietary sugar and dietary fats. Other aspects of what you eat, such as the balance between protein, carbohydrates, and fats in the diet, are also important, but just looking at sugar and fat is a good place to start.

Let's look at sugar first. While fitness, not fat loss, can effectively control the development of insulin resistance and type II diabetes, you can't afford to ignore the effects of the amount of sugar in the diet. One way in which our modern diet conspires to knock our bodies off course is in the amount of simple carbohydrates in our food. Foods high in sugars or simple carbohydrates can suddenly and dramatically affect our blood glucose levels. Our Western-style diet all too often causes us to overdose on sugar, leading to elevated levels of blood glucose. When blood glucose is too high, the pancreas must leap into action and manufacture large quantities of insulin in an effort to bring the sugar levels back in line. Small changes in eating habits can result in big changes in your glucose profile and can save your pancreas and prevent you from developing insulin resistance.

Your body's insulin response to the food you eat depends on how quickly and effectively it can break it down into simple sugars. To compare the effects of different foods, scientists use a method called glycemic index (GI). The glycemic index of foods ranks them in terms of their immediate effect on blood glucose (blood sugar) levels. The quicker foods increase blood glucose levels, the higher the glycemic index number is and the faster the blood sugar response. The glycemic index doesn't depend solely on how much sugar the food contains; it also depends on how it reacts in the body. The presence of fiber, protein, and fat in addition to carbohydrates results in a slower release of carbohydrates into the blood and, hence, a lower glycemic index score.

Recent research has shown that eating a diet rich in foods with low glycemic index scores improves insulin sensitivity.[21] Low glycemic index scores mean a smaller rise in blood sugar, which means that the pancreas doesn't have to produce so much insulin. Furthermore, low–glycemic index diets can help people lose weight and lower blood lipids.

You can use the glycemic index to spare your insulin and boost your energy. According to Patrick Holdford and Judy Ridgway in their book *The Optimum Nutrition Cookbook*, the following guidelines will help you maintain an even glucose profile and spare your pancreas a heavy workload:

- Eat foods with a GI of less than 50 any time.
- Avoid eating foods with a GI higher than 70, unless you eat them with protein foods or with much lower GI foods.
- Consume foods with a GI of between 50 and 70 infrequently or in combination with lower GI foods.

The following table shows the GI scores of some common foods. Note that the scores are based on a comparison to glucose, GI 100, which is the fastest absorbing carbohydrate apart from maltose. If you prefer to use white bread as your standard, simply multiply the numbers in the table by 1.42. For example, glucose would then have a GI of 142. Also note that you might find varying numbers for the same foods in other GI lists. This is because the impact of a food on your blood sugar depends on many factors other than the pure biochemical content of the food such as ripeness, cooking time, fiber and fat content, time of day when eaten, blood insulin levels, and recent activity. Use the GI to make comparisons between food items and to include a greater proportion of foods with a lower GI ranking in your diet.

Glycemic Index of Some Common Food Items

Glycemic Index	Food Lists
Over 70	**Breads:** bagels 72, dark rye bread 76, white bread 72, whole wheat bread 72, waffles 76
	Cereals: Cheerios 74, Corn Bran 75, Corn Chex 83, Crispex 87, Puffed Wheat 90, Rice Chex 89, Rice Krispies 82
	Cookies: graham crackers 74, vanilla wafers 77
	Crackers: Kalvi Norwegian 71, rice cakes 82, saltine 72, water crackers 78
	instant rice 91
	white rice 88
	baked potato 85
	Sweets: jelly beans 80, Life Savers 70
50 to 70	**Breads:** croissant 67, pitta 57, rye bread 64, whole rye 50
	Cereals: Bran Chex 58, Cream of Wheat 66, Frosted Flakes 55, Grapenuts 67, Muesli 60, NutriGrain 66, Shredded Wheat 69, Special K 54, Swiss Muesli 60

Glycemic Index	Food Lists
50 to 70	**Cookies:** oatmeal 55, shortbread 64
	Crackers: rye 63, Stoned Wheat Thins 67
	Desserts: angel food cake 67, blueberry muffin 60, bran muffin 60, danish 59, pound cake 54
	Fruits: apricots canned 64, apricot jam 55, banana 62, canteloupe 65, fruit cocktail 55, mango 55, papaya 58, pineapple 66, raisins 64
	Grains: brown rice 59, cornmeal 68, couscous 65, popcorn 55, sweet corn 55
	sweet potato 54
	orange juice 55
	pasta 68
	honey 58
Under 50	**Beans:** baked beans 43, butter beans 31, chickpeas 33, lentils 30
	pumpernickel bread 49
	Cereals: All Bran 44, oatmeal 49, Rice Bran 19
	Desserts: banana bread 47, fruit bread 47, sponge cake 46
	Fruits: apple 38, apricot, dried 30, cherries 22, grapefruit 25, grapes 43, kiwi 52, orange 43, peach 42, pear 36, plum 24, strawberries 32
	Juices: apple 41, grapefruit 48, pineapple 46
	milk 34, soy milk 31, yogurt 38

Activity 5.3: Am I a Sugar Addict?

This simple quiz will help you determine whether you need to address the issue of sugar in your diet.

1. Do you think about chocolate or sweets all the time and eat them at least once a day?

2. Did your parents give you sweets or chocolate as a child to smooth over emotional upsets?

Activity 5.3. _continued_

3. Do you always keep sweets in the house, in the car, in your desk drawer, or in your backpack or carrying case?

4. Do you expect friends to offer you cake, cookies, or soda pop when you visit?

5. Do you drink more than three sugar-laden soda drinks per week?

6. Do you look at the desserts on a restaurant's menu before you decide on your appetizer and main course?

7. Do you have a favorite store that offers your favorite high–glycemic index foods?

8. Do you feel better after you eat something sweet?

9. Do you ever consume an entire package of cookies or pint of ice cream in one sitting?

10. Do you regularly make a journey or dedicated stop to buy sweets?

If you answered Yes to two or more of these questions, you may have a sugar problem. Activity 5.4 will help you tackle it.

Activity 5.4: Thirteen Simple Ways to Reduce Your Sugar Intake

As you run through this list, put a check mark beside the ones you think you can start doing today to reduce the amount of sugar in your diet:

❑ Don't drink soda or sweetened juice drinks. Their empty calories and sugar content will affect your insulin levels and fat burning.

❑ Dilute fruit juices with water.

❑ Choose a fruit dessert instead of a sugary one.

❑ Read the labels on "low-fat" foods. Avoid ones that use sugar or artificial sweeteners.

❑ Select natural snacks, such as fresh fruit, vegetable sticks, or nuts and raisins instead of cookies and cakes.

❑ Beware of breakfast cereals. Read the labels to find those low in sugar.

❏ When eating out, order a savory starter and skip dessert.

❏ If you must eat something sweet, do so after you have eaten a meal. Then it won't affect your insulin so much.

❏ Stop putting sugar in your tea or coffee.

❏ Eat more whole foods, including whole grains, beans and lentils, and vegetables. Your energy will remain on a more even keel, and you will feel fewer cravings for sugar.

❏ Choose a savory spread instead of jelly for toast.

❏ Watch out for added sugar in otherwise benign foods: Canned carrots often contain sugar, as do some peanut butters, tomato ketchup, sauces for meat, and even salsa dip.

❏ Reduce the sugar in a recipe by about one third. For most recipes, you won't even notice, but your body will thank you.

Exposing the Low Fat Myth

Myth: Low-fat diets lower your chance of getting "clogged arteries."

Fact: You are not what you eat.

Recently, a lot of controversy has erupted over the effectiveness of low-fat diets. Do they, in fact, reduce the risk of arteriosclerosis, or, as some researchers have postulated, do they actually make it worse? To find the answer, we must look at the causes of arteriosclerosis and some of the latest research.

At first, medical researchers thought fatness was a cause of arteriosclerosis. Because they found fat in the arteries of those suffering with the disease, they naturally assumed that people who carried lots of fat in their bodies would most likely accumulate fat in their arteries. That turned out to be dead wrong. After researchers performed autopsies on thousands of dead obese patients over a four-decade period and failed to find a connection between fat in the body and fat in the arteries, they disproved the old theory. One study even found the healthiest arteries in the fattest people.

After failing to link fatness and blocked arteries, scientists turned their attention to diet and fat levels in the blood as the culprit for arteriosclerosis. Cholesterol became the bad guy. This fatlike substance found in foods such as eggs, liver, and kidneys is essential for life because it plays a positive role in healthy cell membranes and essential body processes such as the formation of sex hormones, vitamin D, and bile. Our livers can manufacture all the cholesterol we need. In fact, the body absorbs only about 20 percent of the cholesterol we ingest. The liver makes the rest. However, when scientists dubbed cholesterol the main cause of poor arterial health, doctors encouraged us to eat less of it.

In reality, only a very small percentage of the population, those with abnormal metabolism and very high levels of cholesterol, need to worry about the cholesterol they eat. For the rest of us, only a small percentage of the cholesterol we eat ends up in our blood. In fact, over recent decades, we have reduced our intake of cholesterol, yet our rates of heart disease have increased. Recent research published in the British Medical Journal concluded that despite decades of effort and 31,000 patient-years' worth of data, there is still "only limited and inconclusive evidence" that cutting down on dietary fat has any effect on the risk of heart-related disease and death.[22] As it turns out, it's not so much what we eat that matters, but what our bodies do with what we eat. It's not a case of "you are what you eat," but more a case of "you are what you do about your metabolic and physical fitness."

Between a Rock and a Hard Place: High-Fat and Low-Fat Diets

Little evidence supports the notion that low-fat diets provide any benefit in terms of your blood lipid profile. In fact, evidence exists that eating a low-fat diet can make your blood lipid profile worse. Why? Because low-fat diets tend to be rich in carbohydrates, and they raise insulin levels. Increased insulin levels tend to increase the body's own production of "bad cholesterol."

So what should we be eating, low fat or high fat? The answer to this is "It depends." It depends on *your* physiology. However, a couple of basic rules about fats will help you select a balanced diet that is right for you:

- **Fats don't make you full.** Fats are easier to eat than carbohydrates and proteins. The body is quite good at telling us when we have eaten enough carbohydrates or proteins. On the other hand, we can eat a lot of fat without the body telling us when to apply the brakes. It is too tasty and too nice, and it slides down too easily.
- **Fats are fatter.** Fat is more calorie-dense than carbohydrates and proteins. At 9 calories per gram, as opposed to 4 calories per gram for

carbohydrates and proteins, fat just makes it too easy to take on extra calories without even realizing it.

- **Good fats are good for you.** A diet rich in unsaturated fats, such as nut and seed oils and olive oil, can help raise the levels of "good" cholesterol in the blood.
- **Diets low in fat and very high in carbohydrates are not good.** A diet with very low levels of fat combined with very high levels of carbohydrates results in a decrease in the good cholesterol HDL.

Healthy people eat according to the wisdom of the body, according to appetite, hunger, and satiety signals. You, too, should eat according to your own unique, individual biochemical nature.

Fat Trap: Big Belly Obesity

Do you carry around a big belly? If so, you should know that a lot of fat around the abdomen has been identified as a more important risk factor for cardiovascular disease than the amount of fat, per se. Abdominal fat is visceral fat, fat deposited around the vital organs instead of in specific fat storage areas such as the hips and bottom. You've probably heard the labels "apple-shape" (bad) or "pear-shape" (not so bad). Well, a lot of evidence argues that having a big belly (when your belly measurements are greater than your hip measurement, or being apple-shape) coincides with a poor lipid blood profile. The best way out of this trap? Fitness training. Exercise will do more than a caloric restriction diet to rid you of your abdominal bulge. Dieting may help you lose some weight in the short term, but fitness training will help you change your shape and improve your lipid or fat profile, even if you are still "officially" fat.

National Guidelines on Diet and Exercise

The U.S. and Canadian governments take a very slow and methodical route to modifying their fitness training and nutritional standards. Hence, when they do make a change, it means that a consensus in favor of the change has exceeded resistance to the change. Much of the resistance comes from large, financially powerful special-interest groups and lobbyists for big multinational businesses that take in billions of dollars of profit from our lack of fitness and our increase in fatness. Therefore, I saw it as something of a victory in the battle for good health when, in September 2002, the National Academies' Institute of Medicine for the first time issued new eating and exercise targets aimed at reducing the risk of chronic metabolic diseases.[23] This represents the first major update to the publication of the U.S. Recommended Dietary Allowances since 1989.

The report resulted from a panel of experts who reviewed thousands of scientific studies that link excessive or inadequate eating of fat, carbohydrates, and protein with obesity, heart disease, diabetes, and chronic illness. Recognizing that there is no one right combination for everyone, these new guidelines offer a wide range of nutritional recommendations and a narrow range of exercise recommendations. Good health, they admit, depends on each person's individual biochemistry. The new report stresses flexibility in dietary planning:

- **Exercise:** At least one hour a day of moderate activity is encouraged (heart zones 1 to 3 for both adults and children). This doubles the daily goal set by the 1996 surgeon general's report on the minimum amount of exercise people need.

- **Nutrition:** To meet the daily energy and nutritional requirements of the body while minimizing chronic disease risks, adults should eat within a range of nutrients rather than maintain strict proportions of carbohydrate, protein and fat.

New Dietary Recommendations, from the National Academies' Institute of Medicine

Nutrient or Food Source	Range of Calories for Adults	Range of Calories for Infants and Young Children
Carbohydrates	45 to 65 percent	45 to 65 percent
Fat	20 to 35 percent	25 to 40 percent
Protein	10 to 35 percent	10 to 35 percent

These new guidelines are consistent with the Fit *and* Fat program we have been discussing in this book, and they support the sort of heart zones fitness training I recommend.

Week 4 Summary

I hope you can see now how you can achieve and sustain optimum metabolic fitness at any body weight. Weight loss in itself does not cure metabolic conditions such as insulin resistance, a poor lipid profile, or high blood pressure. You can avoid or reduce all of these conditions and more through metabolic training in heart zones 1 to 3. Fitness, not fat loss, provides the best cure for metabolic diseases. Start your fitness program with metabolic fitness training. It's the place to get the best health benefits, the place to recover, and the place to have fun. Believe me, nothing will make you healthier and happier than the magic of metabolic fitness.

CHAPTER 6

Week 5: Emotional and Physical Fitness Training

Nourishing a Sound Mind in a Sound Body

We are just beginning to realize how intimately the mind and body are connected. Modern science is starting to reveal how our emotional state affects our physical bodies. The effects that we now know are real include how stress can make us fat, how stress can lead to disease and illness, the way in which negative emotions can lead to metabolic disorders, and the link between anger, fear, and heart disease. This week we examine how to counteract the negative effects our stressful lives might be having on our physiology: This is emotional fitness training. After that I go on to talk about physical fitness training or what you can do to increase your heart fitness, flexibility, and strength. First, though, let's take a look at how the different emotional perspectives on aging affected two women.

Is Your Age Influenced by How Old You "Think" You Are? Irene and Lou's Story.

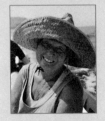

Sixty-five-year-old Irene lives with her small rescue dog, Joseph, in an upstairs apartment in Lands End, San Francisco. She retired five years ago from her job as the administrator of a busy engineering office. Since then, she has seen a dramatic decline in her health. Some would say she's just suffering from "retirement depression," the effect of no longer interacting with 20 people every day, making appointments, fielding telephone calls, locating important papers, fending off difficult clients, and brewing perfect coffee. But it's more than that; Irene sorely misses the former purpose of her life.

Sometimes feelings of loneliness and loss overwhelm her, but Irene has also been noticing physical changes. Her joints are getting stiff and swollen. She can no longer complete the long waterfront walks she and Joseph once loved. Worry about falling has forced her to stop going to the swimming pool for exercise, and a fear of the dark prevents her from going out at night. She spends long winter evenings staring at the television set. Constantly pining for the old hectic days at the office, she now feels old and tired as she waits for a serious illness to strike.

Irene could learn a lot about life from Lou Landreth (pictured on the previous page), who lives on the Mediterranean island of Mallorca. Originally from California, she had sailed her own boat to Mallorca more than 40 years ago with her 1-year-old son. Her long plaited hair, bleached white by the sun and sea, and her tanned, healthy skin give her the look of a Native American matriarch.

After having led a life at sea, Lou settled in the mountains north of the island and became involved in renting holiday properties to tourists. Despite her advancing age, Lou doesn't slow down. Nobody knows her real age (she says she doesn't want to put off any potential boyfriends), but close friends figure she's probably nearly 80. She owns a number of small properties set in olive groves and does the building work mainly on her own, adding a terrace this year, another bedroom the next, hiring labor only when absolutely necessary.

In the summer, she spends her free time rowing her small boat around the dramatic limestone cliffs to collect crabs, lobsters, and other shellfish, sometimes diving down through the clear blue water to capture her prey. In the winter, when the tourists have gone, she swims across the bay, a full mile from headland to headland. She finds the cold, clear water invigorating. Springtime finds Lou heading to the hills. Nobody knows the secret places she visits, or the caves where she sleeps, or even what she eats because she doesn't carry any food. But she comes home happy, the very model of emotional and physical fitness.

What differentiates these two women in their mature years? Irene has allowed her emotional life to affect her physical life. Her feelings about aging and her purpose in life have reduced her willingness to move and engage in physical activity, and that has accelerated the aging process and further physical decline. Her negative emotional state has affected her physical condition. In contrast, Lou refuses to accept old age because she feels there is so much more in life to discover, to live for, and to achieve. She plays a lot, both by herself and with her many friends. Lou listens to her body, and she makes sure her mind never slows her down.

The first step back toward the road to emotional fitness is awareness. Emotional heart zones training is designed to help you become more aware of your emotional state so that you can better manage your emotional life. Many people get stuck in a particular emotion without conscious awareness. When we feel agitated, angry, or stressed, stress hormones flood our bodies like a chemical bath. We need to know how to turn off the tap.

Nourishing the Emotional Heart

Emotional fitness training helps you listen to your emotional heart by becoming aware of your emotional state and learning to shift to a healthier state of mind whenever you slide into a toxic zone. Just as the body heals itself, our emotions can guide us from a condition of stress and poor health to a state of peace, health, and compassion. Peace, health, and compassion are just a few of the benefits of emotional fitness training.

Five emotional heart zones parallel the five physical heart zones. Instead of a range of heart beats, however, the emotional heart zones span a range of emotions that affect the heart and the body. In each zone, the body gains different hormonal, neurological, and biomechanical benefits that influence our level of metabolic and physical fitness. There is a strong connection between our emotional, metabolic, and physical fitness. If you can effectively manage your emotional state by navigating the different emotional zones, you will see results in virtually every aspect of your life.

Take some time to study the emotional heart zones fitness training chart. In which zone do you spend your emotional time?

Each of the five emotional heart zones represents a different state of mind or mood. Just as getting stuck in one physical heart zone limits overall physical fitness, getting stuck in one emotional heart zone limits emotional capacity. Spending time in the top three emotional heart zones—the Safe, Productive, and Performance zones—bestows the most benefits. As you read about emotional zones, ask yourself, "How much time do I spend in this zone?"

Emotional Heart Zones Fitness Training Chart

Zone Number	Emotional Zone	Zone Description—What It Feels Like	Energy or Stress	Zone Result	Long-Term Physiological Result
Zone 1	Safe Zone	Meditative, relaxed, affirming, regenerative, comfortable, compassionate, peaceful	Energy-giving, peace	Energizing Happiness Revitalization	Decreased tiredness. Increased patience, caring, compassion, capacity for love. Improved interpersonal relationships. Better orgasms. Lowered risk of hypertension, type 2 diabetes, immune disorders, and mental disorders. Increased capacity for dealing with pain. Slowing of aging process. Improvement in lung function. Decrease in occurrence of minor disorders such as asthma, irritable bowel syndrome, food intolerance, and skin disorders. Reduced dependence on prescribed medicine. Reduced need for recreational drugs. Improved diet choices.
Zone 2	Productive Zone	High concentration, effective, prolific	Energy-giving	Stimulating Energy-building Satisfaction Increased humor	Improved capacity for undertaking tasks involving mental or physical dexterity. Improved learning ability. Behavior has positive effects on those around you. Highest potential for moments of inspiration or genius.

Zone 3	Performance Zone	Focused, in the flow, "in my element," positive stress, fulfillment, completion	Energy-giving, joy	Achievement Energy gains	Heightened awareness and creativity. Heightened physical endurance and performance. Improved mental performance. Decreased reaction time. Less potential for accidents. Capacity to inspire and energize those around you. Tiring or draining when sustained for long periods.
Zone 4	Distress Zone	Worried, anxious, angry, stressful, scattered, fearful, reactive energy-taking	Cautious, alert	Potentially harmful	Raised blood pressure, bad cholesterol, and increased risk of heart disease. Increased risk of infections, certain cancers, allergies, and autoimmune diseases. Poor concentration leading to heightened risk of accidents and poor learning ability. Poor awareness of others; decline in quality of personal relationships. Increased muscular stress leading to poor posture and even permanent musculoskeletal damage. Hormonal changes that result in weight gain. Increased risk of degenerative disease and premature aging. Reduction in physical functions such as cardiovascular capacity.
Zone 5	Toxic Zone	Out of control, frantic, total panic, disconnected, emergency	Extremely stressful, energy-taking	Toxic: Harms health	Body becomes "maladapted" to stress, leading to permanent health effects. Unhealthful weight gain or weight loss. Heightened susceptibility to mental disorders and addictions. Risk of behavior that damages others.

Zone 1: Safe Zone

The Safe Zone gives us energy. It's where we recharge our batteries, calm ourselves, remain peaceful, and refocus our physical and emotional energy. Your own Safe Zone has unique and personal characteristics. For some, it supports prayer and meditation. For others, music or the sounds of nature create a peaceful inner feeling. A visual memory of a beautiful place or a remembrance of a special moment or thoughts of compassion toward a loved one may ease your heart into the Safe Zone. Just as fitness training strengthens your physical heart, your Safe Zone comforts your emotional heart.

If Zone 1 had a color, it would be blue: a calm and soothing color. Some people find it hard to achieve because it requires calming the mind and focusing energy internally, something our stress-filled, time-starved world makes difficult. But it's worth the effort because it paves the pathway to personal happiness.

Time in the Safe Zone also benefits our metabolic and physical health. Far from compromising our peak metabolic and physical health, it stimulates it. Without harmful hormones and negative messages from the brain, the body can optimize its metabolism and work to improve its physical function. Many studies have demonstrated that such Zone 1 activities as meditation and listening to classical music enhance the immune system, reduce incidence of disease, lower blood pressure, enhance blood chemistry, and generate an overall feeling of well-being.[1]

Zone 2: Productive Zone

The Productive Zone spans a range of feelings that should dominate much of your time at home, work, or play. In Zone 2, you are getting things done and feeling good about yourself and your accomplishments. You feel relatively peaceful and focused as you go about your day-to-day responsibilities. In Zone 2, you enjoy ready and easy access to your emotions and your thoughts.

If Zone 2, the Productive Zone, had a color, it would be green: It facilitates growth of emotional energy, which you can store in your emotional bank account. When you inhabit the green emotional zone, you productively perform tasks that require concentration and attention. All the time you spend there also rewards you physically and metabolically.

Zone 3: Performance Zone

The Performance Zone offers many of the same benefits as Zone 2, with the additional characteristic of even greater focus, concentration, positive intensity, and accomplishment. In it, you strive to achieve peak performance. For example, if you must close a complicated business deal or teach something important to your child, you do it in Zone 3. It accommodates life's big challenges, but it is not a grueling, mind-exhausting, body-breaking space. It is a space full of love and friendship and play as well as hard work.

If Zone 3 had a color, it would be yellow: the color that the leading rider wears in the Tour de France bicycle race, the color that represents the highest emotional level for personal-best performance. You are in this zone if you are working hard but feel in the "flow," in control of events, and if you experience a sense of fulfillment in the moment. You feel alive in every fiber of your being.

Time here also adds to your emotional reservoir, helping you cope with life's inevitable crises. It also adds tremendously to your metabolic and physical health.

Zone 4: Distress Zone

Zone 4 drains us of energy. It's where bad emotional stuff starts to happen and we can do stupid things we later regret. In it swirl feelings of fear, worry, anger, anxiety, depression, desperation, guilt, and helplessness. When circumstances trigger the body's stress response, the resultant physiological changes begin to adversely affect heart rate, blood chemistry, and activity in all the cells and organs of the body. High emotional tension taxes metabolic and physical health.

If Zone 4, the Distress Zone, had a color, it would be orange: the color of a warning signal. In the Distress Zone, you find it harder to think clearly as your emotions begin to take over from your rational mind. In Zone 4, we become much less productive in our work and much more destructive in our relationships. When you hear yourself saying to yourself or others, "I feel stressed out," or your blood pressure or heart rate tell you so, you're spending too much of your time in the orange zone. Because this zone robs energy from your emotional bank account, decreasing your motivation, reducing your productivity, and preventing you from feeling the joy that should dominate your life, it ends up hurting your physical and metabolic health.

Zone 5: Toxic Zone

Stay out of the Toxic Zone. Here you are emotional redlining, pressing your foot on the pedal of emotional catastrophe. When you go out of control emotionally, you cannot think rationally; you react to situations and people with aggression, violence, and hysteria. Time in the red zone leads to abusive and destructive behavior. It is a toxic state, not only damaging the person experiencing Zone 5, but also threatening to the welfare of anyone else nearby. Stay out of it yourself, but also avoid people who spend time there.

If Zone 5, the Toxic Zone, had a color, it would be red: the color of danger. It is as toxic and corrosive as battery acid. Few people can pull themselves out of it all by themselves, and they must turn to mental health professionals to guide them back to the lower zones. If you spend any time in Zone 5, you will lose a lot of energy as it drains you of positive feelings, understanding, and appreciation, and leaves you in a state of panic and frantic metabolic and physical symptoms.

The Mind-Body Connection

The brain and the body influence each other in mysterious ways. Our emotions and perceptions of our world cause our brain to send messages that affect heart rate, blood chemistry, and the activity of every cell in the body. A positive interpretation of the world around us affect our bodies positively, while bad feelings about our environment, such as stress, affect our bodies negatively.

Our thoughts and feelings influence the body via the nervous and the circulatory systems. The brain sends nerve impulses into all of the body's tissues, influencing their behavior. The brain affects the immune system with nerve endings extending into the bone marrow (the birthplace of all white cells), the thymus, the spleen, and the lymph nodes. It also reaches into all the glands of the endocrine system, all the bones, the muscles, all the internal organs, and even the walls of the veins and arteries. Its signals thus affect how the heart functions.

The brain is also a gland, manufacturing thousands of different chemicals and releasing them into the bloodstream, ultimately reaching and influencing all the body's tissues. The brain is a 24-hour-a-day drugstore, producing many more drugs than science will ever invent. Finally, it's a two-way street. The body sends its own signals to the brain.

Arresting the Stress Monster

Stress comes in many forms. Physical stress taxes the muscles; emotional stress taxes the mind. Stress can be positive and can be negative, depending our interpretation and response to it. It can give us energy, and it can take it away. Negative emotional response to stress, the sort that occurs in emotional heart zones 4 and 5, is a huge energy drain, while a positive emotional response to stress, the sort that occurs in emotional heart zones 1 to 3, is a big energy builder.

While all of us experience a full range of emotions in our lives, most people operate within a familiar set of feelings day in and day out. When we carry positive emotions within us, our heart gets healthier; when we carry negative or energy-draining emotions with us, our heart suffers. For most everyone, certain triggering situations can cause us to shift out of the lower emotional zones and into the higher ones. For example, some people habitually react to almost any situation with emotions of fear and worry, never seeing a silver lining in any of life's dark clouds. Others seem addicted to redlining with rage or panic. These emotions can be triggered instantly at home or at work when different challenges or crises arise. Conversely, some folks maintain a sunny disposition throughout even the most stressful situations, finding a silver lining in every dark cloud. By responding to challenging, stressful situations with positive emotional energy, the heart muscle gets stronger and fitter, and so does our emotional fitness. Believe it or not, you can emotionally train for it.

Healthy people stay in touch with their emotions and actively express and share what they feel. By actively using energy-giving emotions, you get stronger and healthier in much the same way as energy-giving activities make your physical heart stronger and healthier. The benefits of energy-giving emotional fitness? One word: *happiness*. You are never too fat to deny yourself happiness and all the other benefits of emotional fitness. Thinness does not make you happy, or benefit your emotional fitness. Everyone can learn to control their emotions and to not allow their emotions to control them. Emotional fitness training involves activities that lead to energy-giving and an increase in positive feelings and confidence in abilities. It all happens in the three lower emotional heart zones.

When you get emotionally fit, you can visit the bottom three emotional heart zones whenever you choose, entering emotional Zone 1 to re-energize yourself, settling into emotional Zone 2 to get things done, and moving into emotional Zone 3 when a challenging task presents itself. You recognize the caution signs that tell you you're getting into Zone 4, and you manage to deal with your feelings and bring yourself down from the distress zone. You never, ever let yourself slide into toxic Zone 5.

Emotional fitness not only affects how we feel and how we interact with our colleagues, friends, and lovers, but it also influences how well our bodies actually function. For years, mainstream medicine did not accept the mind-body link, dismissing it as nonscientific and, therefore, not reliable. Today, however, scientific evidence has changed that opinion. Energy-taking emotions really do harm human health. For example, an accumulation of stressful events in our lives, such as financial difficulties, the death of a pet or loved one, conflict with a parent or child, or a crisis at work, causes a host of physiological and biochemical changes. Scientists call this the "stress response." It is the cascading of internal bodily changes that result from a dose of chemical, hormonal, and neural reactions to stress. Typical stress responses include nervous tension, upset stomach, and changes in weight, particularly weight gain.

Isn't that interesting? Stress makes us fat. The stress response not only robs us of good health, but it contributes to obesity. As negative stress piles up, the body responds with lethargy. It's just too much trouble to move. Lack of energy results in lack of exercise and physical activity, often resulting in fat gain. Stress also makes us eat in a disordered and self-destructive way, choosing foods for emotional reasons rather than nutritional ones. Eating may calm emotions, because eating for emotional satisfaction makes us feel better, but that's a dangerous way to cheer yourself up: In the long run, it makes you feel worse as you get more fat and less fit.

Activity 6.1: Completing Your Emotional Checkup

In the previous chapters, we touched on the importance of living an emotionally fit life. You've completed a number of emotional fitness-related activities, and you may have found some aspects of the Fit *and* Fat Personal Activity Program emotionally demanding. Actually, I've urged you to make quite a few emotional fitness changes already. Now it's time to put it all together, administering a thorough emotional fitness checkup to identify areas where you need to work harder to gain and sustain emotional fitness.

This exercise will help you set your emotional heart zones goals. First review the notes you made in your personal fitness log for Activities 2.1, 2.6, 2.7, and 2.8. Next, work through the following self-assessments, looking for emotional road blocks for any emotional areas of your life that could be holding you back.

As you complete the following three self-assessments, remember that a sense of humor is a sure sign of emotional health. Use humor for emotional support as you take these assessments. We'll examine the results and what they mean after you've completed all these assessments.

Self-Assessment A: Identifying Anxiety and Self-Defeating Beliefs

Purpose: To obtain a current reading on your emotional fitness and to assist in setting your emotional heart zone goals.

Scoring: Circle the following statements according to a range from 1 (not true at all) to 5 (very true).

Statement	Not True	→	Very True
1. You must always have love and approval.	1 2	3	4 5
2. You must always prove to be thoroughly competent, adequate, and achieving.	1 2	3	4 5
3. Misery comes from external pressures.	1 2	3	4 5
4. If something seems fearsome, you must preoccupy yourself with it and make yourself anxious.	1 2	3	4 5
5. The past remains all important.	1 2	3	4 5

Score: _____ (the sum of the numbers)

Self-Assessment B: Detecting Emotional Patterns

Purpose: To understand your emotional habits in order to determine how you can better manage them.

Scoring: Rate how often you experience each emotion by circling the number that best expresses your tendency to engage in it.

Emotion	Rarely	→	Very Often
1. Worry	1 2	3	4 5
2. Fear	1 2	3	4 5
3. Anger	1 2	3	4 5
4. Depression	1 2	3	4 5

Score: _____ (the sum of the numbers)

Activity 6.1. *continued*

Self-Assessment C: Emotional Strength

Purpose: To obtain a current reading on your emotional strengths in order to better understand how to make them stronger.

Scoring: To obtain a current reading on your emotional strengths in order to better understand how to make them stronger.

Description	Often True → Seldom True
1. Awareness of others' feelings	1 2 3 4 5
2. Self-control, ability to manage your emotions effectively	1 2 3 4 5
3. Self-motivation	1 2 3 4 5
4. Harmonious relationships at home and work	1 2 3 4 5
5. Self-awareness of your own feelings at any given moment	1 2 3 4 5

Score: _____ (the sum of the numbers)

What Do Your Friends Think?

While you can learn a lot when you assess your own emotional fitness, you can learn even more when you get feedback from people who know you well. You can make copies of this questionnaire and ask friends, loved ones, or colleagues to fill them out as honestly as they can. Compare how others view you with how you view yourself. The truth probably rests between these two viewpoints.

Analyzing Your Level of Emotional Fitness

You can use the information derived from your emotional checkup to strengthen yourself emotionally. As you filled out the self-assessments, did you notice anything that might prompt you to make some changes? Just an inkling of new awareness can help you begin the journey toward greater health and happiness. Add a little desire and motivation, and you can take the first positive steps in that direction.

Interpreting Your Anxiety and Self-Defeating Beliefs: Self-Assessment A

A higher score (16 to 26) means that you tend to put a lot of pressure on yourself and dismiss whatever you do as never enough. You may be holding yourself back, making yourself a hostage of your negative emotional energy. Do you sometimes feel like a frightened child who goes to bed burdened with all your faults and having heard a scary story just before bedtime? Fear and anxiety like that make our hearts beat faster as our bodies pour stress hormones into our systems. A lower score (5 to 15) means you can seize more control over the way you want to live your life and the things you want for yourself instead of giving up that power to others or to your past.

If your score was high, you might begin loving yourself more by making regular statements of compassion like these:

1. I value all the love and approval I receive.
2. I am competent and adequate.
3. I can control the amount of pressure in my life.
4. If something frightens me, I can calm and protect myself.
5. I accept this moment and this day as a gift.

Remind yourself of the old saying: "The past is history, the future is a mystery, today is a gift, and that's why they call it the present."

Analyzing Your Emotional Patterns: Self-Assessment B

Most of us tend to rely heavily on certain emotions. Our particular emotional patterns develop each time the response to an emotional stimulus is reinforced. For instance, if people applaud you for reacting to an aggressive person with diplomacy, you will tend to rely on that response in difficult situations. Once you understand your emotional pattern, you can do more to apply, manage, or change that habit.

The four emotions from Self-Assessment B—worry, fear, anger, and depression—are certainly valid emotions in our lives, but they are not the ones we should let guide us. These emotions work in our favor only when they motivate us to action when exposed to physical danger or a threat to our well-being. Without danger, they are not healthy emotional patterns. In inappropriate situations, these emotions become dangers themselves as they propel us into the Distress Zone.

Compassion provides the best antidote. If you scored high (11 to 20) on Self-Assessment B, you earn an extra dose of compassion. Looking back over your life, can you spot events, perhaps painful ones to recall, that aroused feelings of worry, fear, anger, or depression? For example, if you grew up in an abusive environment,

---

Activity 6.1. *continued*

you may find yourself reacting today with the same emotions that swept over you then. They can so easily be triggered by events in your adult life. Some emotions, however, spring not from your personal history, but from a biochemical source, such as an insufficient release of certain natural hormones. That's the case with severe depression. Extreme cases of worry, fear, anger, and depression require psychiatric treatment and possibly medication to counteract real biochemical imbalances.

A lower score on this self-assessment means you spend more time in zones 1, 2, and 3 than in Zone 4, which is good. A low score also means you have more room in your life for happiness, contentment, and love. You more often use worry, anger, fear, and depression to stimulate prompt and necessary corrections.

Recognizing Your Emotional Strengths: Self-Assessment C

We can all benefit from greater emotional strength. The most important emotional strength is a keen awareness of your own feelings at any given moment. Tuning in to your emotional feelings will guide you toward becoming emotionally stronger. Awareness of the feelings of others and compassion for these feelings put you in a position to interact and connect with others in a positive way. A high score (16 to 25) on this self-assessment means that these qualities need more attention and development. You might consider starting to do so by making a conscious effort at various times throughout your day to take stock of your feelings. Take a few deep breaths and ask yourself "How am I feeling right now?" Just by asking the question, you are speaking to and listening to your emotional heart. And conversations with your emotional heart automatically strengthen it. Your emotional heart works on the same principle as your physical heart: Use it or lose it.

Share the conversations you conduct with your emotional heart. Present them to others in a sincere and caring way. Invite them to do the same. Each time you connect with someone important to you, ask the question "What and how are you feeling today or at this moment?" At first it may seem somewhat trite, but when you do it in a heartfelt manner, you will rejoice at the connection between your two hearts. Make eye contact. The eyes are not only the windows to the soul, but they are also the windows to the heart. When you make eye contact with another person, you increase the chance of making heart connection.

The preceding activity should have helped you pinpoint some areas in your emotional life that you would like to improve. For instance, do you want to pay more attention to your anxiety and self-defeating beliefs? To your emotional patterns? To your emotional strengths? Whatever area you identified the following activity will assist you in finding an emotional fitness training activity that will mitigate some of the physical affects your emotional life may be having.

Activity 6.2: Identifying Your Emotional Fitness-Training Activities

The following is a list of the possible emotional areas that you may have identified in the previous activity as a priority for you to work on. Next to each emotional area are some ideas for emotional fitness training activities that you could build into your training program to counter bad emotions and replace them with better ones.

Emotional Area	Emotional Fitness Training Activity
Certain daily situations or people elicit from me the same negative response.	Try to identify and understand why this emotional response may be happening. When did you develop that pattern of behavior? How can you break out of that cycle? Use your friends or a professional to help you if you get stuck.
I often feel stressed out.	Try to pace yourself, and don't set your goals too high or too unrealistically. Practice saying "no" to additional demands on your time. Spend time each day in Zone 1, the Safe Zone, to regenerate. Promise yourself that you will meditate, listen to music, or use prayer at least 20 minutes each day.
Aggravations ignite my anger more often than I'd like.	Take a class or a home-study course that teaches you new ways to cope with stress. The moment you notice a negative "mood shift," award yourself a timeout and converse with your heart muscle to calm yourself. Then consciously shift down from Zone 4 to Zone 1 or Zone 2.
I suffer from too much anxiety and too many self-defeating beliefs.	Practice compassion with yourself and others. Understanding and forgiveness heal most emotional wounds. Define yourself as a good person, and congratulate yourself on all your accomplishments.

Activity 6.2. *continued*

Worry, fear, anger, and depression bother me a lot.	These emotions are designed to draw our attention to things that need to be addressed in our lives. Try to identify the underlying reasons for these emotions, and take a practical approach to focusing on the things that you want in your life rather than what you want to get rid of.
I want to change some of my emotional patterns.	Relearn new patterns by reinforcing different behaviors. For example, after your workday, instead of watching television, join a club and take a fitness training class.
I want to develop emotional awareness.	Focus on becoming more emotionally aware by slowing down your activities and spending more energy on noticing. Each time you connect with someone, look into that person's eyes and ask how he or she is feeling. Try to be "present" with every person you interact with.

When you have chosen some new emotional fitness-training activities, put them into daily practice. Practice may not make you perfect, but it will help you replace unwanted habits with those that will make you more emotionally fit and, most important, happier.

Physical Fitness Training

Now that we've explored one side of the mind-body connection, it's time to look at the other side, the physical fitness side. The key components of physical fitness are listed here:

- Cardiovascular fitness
- Muscular strength
- Flexibility

The training for these components includes the following:

- **Cardiovascular training.** This includes movement activities that cause your heart rate to increase into the physical heart zones, to make the heart and lungs healthier.

- **Muscular strength training.** This involves the use of resistance activities to stimulate muscles in order to make them stronger.
- **Flexibility training.** This stretches the muscles to make them longer and improve their range of motion.

No single training activity provides you with each of these three types of workouts, although some modern exercise classes do give you a mix of all three within the allotted class time of, say, 60 minutes.

Benefits of the Three Key Components of Physical Fitness

Cardiovascular Training	Muscular Strength Training	Flexibility Training
The heart becomes stronger, which means that it takes fewer beats to pump the same amount of blood.	Muscle fibers become stronger, giving you more strength.	Muscles elongate, which increases muscle strength with a greater range of motion.
The heart becomes bigger, which means that it can pump more blood with each contraction.	Muscles increase in size, giving you more muscle fibers and more strength.	Muscle tension is reduced, which can lead to quicker recovery between workouts.
The body develops more blood capillaries, which means that blood can get to the tissues more easily.	The fuel-burning capacity within muscles is improved, enhancing the body's fat-burning ability.	Muscle balance improves, leading to better posture and fewer injuries.
The enzymes that facilitate fuel burning increase their efficiency, which means that the body burns more fat and can exercise for longer without tiring.	The joints receive improved support from surrounding muscles, decreasing risk of injury.	Low-back problems are prevented.
Depression and anxiety are lowered, stress is relieved, and mood states are improved.	Bones become denser, reducing the risk of broken bones and osteoporosis, particularly as age progresses.	Functional capacity is maintained.

Benefits of the Three Key Components of Physical Fitness *continued*

Cardiovascular Training	Muscular Strength Training	Flexibility Training
Body shape improves, leading to improved body image.	Body shape improves, leading to improved body image.	Energy level and outlook on life improve.
Efficiency in sports improves as endurance and speed increase.	Efficiency in sports improves as strength increases.	Muscle elasticity improves, adding to agility and speed.
Risk of cardiovascular disease, diabetes, and some types of cancers decreases.	Posture improves and risk of postural-related injuries decreases.	Posture improves, which enhances personal appearance.

Cardiovascular Training

Cardiovascular training is just that: training for the heart (cardio) and blood vessels (vascular) that deliver nutrients throughout the body. A basic cardiovascular workout has a beginning (a warm-up), a middle (in which you continuously raise your heart rate), and an end (the cool-down). If you were to plot your heart rate in beats per minute for an entire workout period, it would look like the next figure.

The warm-up and cool-down periods are important because you need to give your system a chance to prepare for the middle or main set of the workout and to recover from it. To get the most out of any training activity, you need a sound plan for the workout: what to do, the *mode* of exercise; how many times a week, the *frequency;* how long you have to do it, the *duration;* and how hard you do it, the *intensity.*

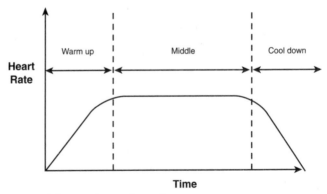

A basic cardiovascular workout.

Mode

Any exercise that increases your heart rate sufficiently is, by definition, cardio-vascular training. If you choose fitness-training activities that use large groups of muscles—for example, your thighs, buttocks, and lower back in stair climbing—you'll be able to sustain the exercise for a longer period. You can't sustain lifting weights above your head for long because you use just an isolated group of muscles. In general, the best workouts for cardiovascular conditioning are activities like walking, running, swimming, skating, cycling, rowing, cross-country skiing, stepping, and snowshoeing.

Frequency and Duration

As a rule of thumb, the more frequently you engage in cardiovascular training and the more time you invest in it, the more benefits you get. By increasing exercise frequency, you realize improved circulation and better burning of fuels for some time after you have ceased the activity. Some recent research indicates that three 10-minute bouts of exercise per day may be more beneficial than one 30-minute bout.[2] However, in terms of fat burning improvements (and I'll talk more about this in the next chapter), longer training time periods offer more rewards because there is a gradual shift to greater dependence on fat burning during the longer workout.

Just as no one fitness program fits all, no firm guidelines on frequency and duration will suit everybody. You must judge how your body feels and how it responds to exercise. However, you will want to think about the following pointers as you set about designing your own optimum plan:

- The amount of warm-up time differs from person to person. Depending on your targeted heart zone for each specific workout, you may need to vary your warm-up time. For example, my friend Paul, age 85, needs about 10 minutes of walking before he can run comfortably.

- Where you work out might dictate the length of your workout. If you drive to your health club, change into workout clothes when you arrive, and shower afterward, it's probably more convenient to do a single 30-minute workout than 3 different training sessions each for 10 minutes. On the other hand, if you can integrate cardiovascular training into your daily activities, you can accumulate benefits by walking to work, walking up and down stairs whenever possible, and stretching when forced to wait.

  Can you incorporate fitness training into your daily routine? One friend of mine works at a large airplane manufacturing site that sprawls two miles from one end of the plant to the other. By using his bike instead of the electric golf cart the company provides, he accumulates 4 to 6 bouts of 10 minutes of additional exercise each workday.

- The recovery time between workouts is vital: You need to recover fully between workouts in order to gain optimum benefits. Knowing whether you have fully recovered is a key skill in your becoming an athlete. You can gauge it by measuring your heart rate and by sensing your energy levels. Your recovery capability will improve as you get fitter. Listen to your body. Recognize its signals.

How Do I Know If I've Recovered?

You are ready to exercise again when ...
- You feel like exercising again and look forward to it.
- You feel full of energy.
- Your resting and delta heart rates are back to normal.
- Your heart rate increases gradually rather than quickly when you start exercising again.
- Your muscles feel strong and supple with no soreness.

Rest and recover when ...
- You feel stale and do not look forward to training.
- You are uninterested in exercise.
- You lack energy.
- You feel tired.
- Your muscles feel weak, sore, or stiff.
- You sense that you are ill or injured.

Intensity

I cannot prescribe an intensity level for you. You must figure it out for yourself. In the past, experts prescribed exercise intensity levels of 70 to 85 percent of the maximum heart rate. Yes, that might be right for some people, but not for anyone just starting out on a cardiovascular program. Recent research has shown that untrained athletes gain cardiovascular benefits at only 50 to 60 percent of their maximum heart rate.[3] For the unfit, a Zone 2 workout might be too hard. As a basic guide, consider these guidelines to select the right exercise intensity:

- **Talk test.** The exercise intensity should not prevent you from talking while you are training. If you gasp for air between words and feel "winded," reduce the intensity.

- **Sustainability.** You should be exercising at an intensity at which you feel you can keep going for a sustained period of time. If you find yourself looking toward the next lamppost when you're jogging, you're probably going too hard. Ease off until you feel you can keep going without concentrating on it too much.

Zone 3 intensity suits most moderately fit people. If you are new to physical training or haven't done any for a while, you may want to work out in zones 1 or 2 for a time. If so, monitor how you feel; after only a couple weeks of training, you should be ready to move up a zone but still pass the talk test and the sustainability test.

If you are ready to learn the advanced version of finding the right intensity for your workouts, then read this section. What the talk test and the sustainability test are actually doing is helping you to find your aerobic level of training. *Aerobic* literally means "with oxygen," and it's the state at which the body uses oxygen to metabolize energy. As you increase your exercise intensity, you reach a point called the anaerobic threshold, at which the body can no longer deliver sufficient oxygen to the muscles in the quantities they need to metabolize energy aerobically. At this point, the muscles turn to a backup plan for making energy via the anaerobic metabolism.

Whereas aerobic metabolism relies mostly on fat for energy, anaerobic relies mostly on sugar for energy. Because we have a lot of fat in our bodies, we can keep our aerobic system going for a long time. If we rely solely on the anaerobic system (at very high intensity levels), not only does our energy store run out quickly because we are exhausting limited sugar supplies, but our bodies create a lactic acid waste product. Lactic acid buildup has a crippling effect on the muscles, cramping them up and forcing us to stop the exercise. Although you can gain great benefits from training anaerobically, which I discuss more thoroughly in Chapter 7, you will focus for now on those you get when you train aerobically.

How I Discovered the Benefits of Aerobic Training: Lorraine's Story

Just as Lorraine discovered the specific benefits of metabolic training in the low zones, she also discovered the particular changes that are stimulated by Zone 3 training. Here she tells us about her experience with running and Zone 3.

Even before I knew about heart zone training, I had purchased a heart rate monitor and was using it a lot. I didn't really understand the best way to use it, so I asked a trainer at my local fitness club to help me. She recommended that I run on the treadmill at a heart rate up to 168. I told her I was not a running sort of person. I actually hated running. I found it awkward and painful, and it made me feel ungainly. She encouraged me to start off with just 5 minutes and then build up to 15. Reluctantly, I agreed to give it a shot.

Determined to get the benefits of fitness, I made myself go through the running part of my training program. The running was so hard—my heart was pounding out of my chest, and my legs felt heavy and stiff afterward. I was so focused on the clock and my heart rate monitor the whole time that I was counting down the seconds of each minute I had to stay there with various parts of my body flapping around in all directions. Thank goodness I always did the workout in the early morning when the gym was nearly empty!

Then I attended a Heart Zones Training Seminar and learned about individual maximum heart rates and Zone 3, the Aerobic Zone. According to this new information, the best aerobic heart rate range for me was down around 133 to 148, not way up at 168. I decided to try out the new heart rates for running, just to see what happened. Up to that point, I had been doing my 15 minutes of running for about 6 weeks and had seen no improvement in the distance I could run or in my heart rate over that 15 minutes.

Running at the new aerobic level had a totally different feel. I no longer found myself fixated on the clock, but I was able to watch the morning news on the overhead monitors and even talk to my neighbor. The minutes flew by. It was no longer "dreadmill," as I had coined it. By lowering my running speed to maintain this new heart rate, after three days I found that I could increase a little bit. After two weeks, I noticed a huge change: I was back to running the same distance as when I was running at 168, but now I was maintaining a heart rate of just 148. Before, I had been training anaerobically, above my body's capacity for adaptation. Now, training aerobically, I realized the cardiovascular benefits I was seeking.

Of course, the anaerobic threshold varies for each individual. In a recent study of obese subjects, researchers found their anaerobic threshold to be, on average, 78 percent of their maximum heart rate, plus or minus 6 percent.[4] That might not sound like a big variance, but for a person with a maximum heart rate of 180, the anaerobic threshold could fall anywhere between 130 and 150 bpm.

It's important for you to determine your own anaerobic threshold because it serves as a key indicator of fitness: the higher, the better. Also, for people concerned with fat burning or endurance training, the point just below the anaerobic threshold represents the heart rate at which we can burn total calories and fat at the highest possible rate and keep going. If we want to burn more fat and more calories, we not only want to find this point, but we also want to raise it by getting fitter. I'll talk more about this in Chapter 7, where you will find out how to determine your anaerobic threshold heart rate number. For now, you need only a rough idea of it. With careful observation and by listening to your body, you can determine that rough number. Use the following guidelines for now, and then take the anaerobic threshold test in Chapter 7 later. Note your heart rate number at which ...

- Your training intensity causes you to fail the talk test.
- Your training intensity causes you to fail the sustainability test.

You can also record the highest heart rate you can sustain for several minutes while working out vigorously. Pay attention to the "turning point" in your tolerance to increased exercise intensity (that is, the moment when, having increased your heart rate up through the zones, you suddenly feel as though you really can't boost it further).

Maintaining a constant intensity in your cardiovascular training is called a steady state workout and is fine, but variety adds enjoyment. For example, a crisscross workout would involve moving back and forth between the floor of one zone and the ceiling of another; a workout plan is provided in Activity 6.3.

During a cardiovascular workout, you aim to spend most of the time in your aerobic heart rate range, but you can derive additional benefits by exceeding your sustainable heart rate for a few minutes and then dropping down to a lower heart rate to recover. This is called interval training, a routine that, over time, pushes up your anaerobic threshold. An example of an interval workout is given in Chapter 7.

Activity 6.3: Cardiovascular Crisscross Workout

This is a workout you can do inside or outside. You actually crisscross two zones, zones 2 and 3. Throughout the workout, you'll be either increasing your heart rate or allowing it to drop—you never stay at a steady heart rate, so you'll be watching your heart rate monitor closely. Write in your own heart rate numbers before you start the workout. Your heart rate should follow the profile in the following figure.

Elapsed Time (Min)	Workout Plan	Heart Zone	Your Heart Rate (bpm)	Interval Time (Min)
0 to 5	Warm up to the bottom of Z2.	2	_____	5
5 to 8	Increase HR to bottom of Z3.	3	_____	3
8 to 11	Increase HR to top of Z3.	3	_____	3
11 to 14	Recover to bottom of Z2.	2	_____	3
14 to 17	Increase HR to top of Z3.	3	_____	3
17 to 20	Recover to bottom of Z2.	2	_____	3
20 to 23	Increase HR to top of Z3.	3	_____	3
23 to 26	Recover to bottom of Z2.	2	_____	3
26 to 29	Increase HR to top of Z3.	3	_____	3
29 to 32	Recover to bottom of Z2.	2	_____	3
32 to 35	Increase HR to top of Z3.	3	_____	3
35 to 38	Recover to bottom of Z2.	2	_____	3
38 to 41	Increase HR to top of Z3.	3	_____	3
41 to 45	Cool down to bottom of Z2 and then Z1.	2 1	_____	4

Heart rate plot of the cardiovascular crisscross workout.

Muscular Strength Training

Everyday activities require a certain amount of muscular strength and endurance—even routine tasks such as lifting children, doing yard work and housework, and washing the car. The same is true in the workplace, whether you do any heavy lifting or not. By gaining muscular strength, we become healthier. For those who suffer from back pain, specific strength-training activities can help reduce or eliminate the pain. By maintaining your muscle strength, you will also suffer fewer injuries and maintain your muscle power as you age. For women, strength or resistance training helps preserve bone mass and prevent osteoporosis. Think of strength training as investing in a personal health insurance policy.

Strength training also leads to increases in metabolic rate, which is primarily determined by your lean body mass: The more muscle mass you have, the more calories you burn even when you're sleeping. For example, a decrease in your body fat of 2 percent, coupled with an increase in muscle mass of 5 percent, will not only make you look healthier, but it will also boost your resting metabolism by 10 to 15 percent. As with cardiovascular training, you achieve such a muscular training goal with activities that suit your special situation, which dictates the mode, frequency, duration, and intensity of the workout.

Mode

Must you go to the gym to resistance train? Not necessarily. Remember, strength training is anything that loads and overloads your skeletal muscles. Any activity which gives additional load to your muscles can give you a strength workout. For example, a very unconditioned athlete might use walking up a flight of stairs as an initial strength-training activity. As you progress, you may find it easier to go to a health club, with people and equipment to help you get a good workout. If you participate in a particular sport, you may opt for sport-specific strength training, such as the use of hand paddles while swimming. Whatever the case, mull over these ideas for incorporating strength training into your routine.

The following are some outdoor ideas:

- If you walk, introduce walking up hills.
- If you run, do hill repeats.
- Some municipal parks maintain outdoor circuits that you can incorporate into your walk or run.
- Walk or run up steps.
- If you cycle, climb hills.
- Walk through deep snow (or, better yet, shovel some).

- Carry a pack when hiking.
- Try cross-country or downhill skiing.
- Take up rock climbing.

Or try these athletic club ideas:

- Do indoor cycling using a high resistance.
- Exercise using a box step.
- Increase the resistance on a rowing machine.
- Increase the elevation or resistance on a cardio machine, like an elliptical trainer.
- Join a strength-training exercise class.
- Work out with free weights.
- Investigate Swiss ball (a large air-filled rubber ball you can sit on to perform exercises) training.
- Try Pilates and certain types of yoga workouts.
- Attend parent and baby classes using the baby's weight as resistance.

Here are some home exercise ideas:

- Augment home routines using exercise bands or small weights.
- Look into home video routines, available for a whole variety of movement activities.

Once you've added some resistance elements to your daily activities or workouts, you'll want to determine how often you can or should do them.

Frequency

Strength training follows the basic Law of Diminishing Returns: Doing a little gets you a lot, but doing too much gets you less. With strength training, the more you do, the less you benefit as you increase it more and more. The initial training session gives you the most. As a matter of fact, a little *can be* better than a lot. *A lot of strength training may give you maximum benefits, but not optimum benefits.* People who have led fairly inactive lives obtain the greatest benefits from initiating a training program. Surprisingly, perhaps, they'll realize a much greater health benefit than the already fit individual who trains even more hours. Sure, the extra few hours of fitness training might result in some improvement, but not the massive health improvements a sedentary person will see.

Duration and Intensity

If you've never done any strength training, you should proceed cautiously. It's easy to overdo it and end up hurting rather than helping yourself, particularly when you are lifting weights. In terms of knowing how much weight to lift, you've hit the right intensity when you can "feel" your muscles the next day but can't sense any soreness. You can find this level only through trial and error. After you warm up adequately, see what maximum weight you can lift for one repetition. Then use 60 to 70 percent of that amount, lifting smoothly and slowly.

The following basic guidelines will help you get the most from using resistance machines:

- Do 5 to 10 minutes of light cardiovascular activity in zones 1 or 2 before lifting weights.
- Do a set of 10 to 12 repetitions.
- Do two to three sets per activity per workout.
- Keep track of the amount that you are lifting or doing.
- Lift for both the lower body and the upper body in one session if you are doing resistance training two times per week.

Strength training boosts energy. After the workout, you should feel good, even joyful. Because you increase your energy by using your muscles to get stronger, you'll relish the emotional feeling you get from the workout as much as the physical feeling. Weight lifters often say, "Use it or lose it." To put it another way, "Use energy to gain energy."

A few simple reminders will help you enjoy your strength-training program, eliminate muscle soreness, and keep yourself safe and injury-free:

- Warm up before any resistance exercise, and cool down afterward.
- For both safety and injury prevention, pay attention to proper technique and form.
- Exercise large muscles before tackling small muscle groups.
- Breathe in a steady, continuous fashion while performing lifts. Do not hold your breath; this results in an increase in blood pressure and reduces the return of blood to the heart.
- Overcome plateaus in training by adding variability to your training with recovery periods, cross-training, and different routines.

I meet a lot of people, many of them women, who misunderstand resistance training because they believe some of the myths and propaganda that surrounds it. They think of it as bodybuilding. It's not. Forgive me for climbing on my soapbox for a minute, but I really must set the record straight by exposing the myths:

Myth: Strength training, especially for women, results in big muscles.

Reality: This is very rarely true. You have to work really hard as a female to build large-looking muscles. You will first tone and strengthen your current muscle mass.

Myth: Strength training increases cardiovascular ability.

Reality: Strength training does not greatly improve cardiovascular ability.

Myth: It takes a long time to get results from strength training.

Reality: For the unfit, strength gains occur very quickly. This rapid improvement often results in motivation that keeps you on the program.

Myth: Men gain strength faster than women.

Reality: Women gain strength just as quickly as men for the first 12 weeks. However, men generally increase their muscle size more than women do.[5]

Myth: Strength training can hurt your sport-specific training and decrease your performance.

Reality: By adding strength training to your fitness program, you'll get more from your sport-specific workouts and enhance your performances.

Activity 6.4: Starting a Strength-Training Program

First assess your current level of fitness and your strength-training habits, if any. Have you done strength training before? Do you need to learn more about strength training? What facilities do you have available? Place yourself somewhere in the following list of strength-training levels to see what activities to try.

I've never done any strength training.

- Try sport-specific training, such as walking, strength running, or cycling up hills.
- Join a class in which an instructor guides you through a strength-training routine. Depending on your level of fitness, this could be Pilates, aqua aerobics, or "Hot Iron" (a group exercise class set to music in which each person lifts a weighted bar). Work with the instructor to ensure the right level for you.

I've done some, but I've never kept it up.

- Try some different ideas, such as purchasing some elastic exercise bands and learning how to use them and then finding a time of day and place where you can carry out a program.

- Experiment with a new method of strength training, such as Swiss ball (a method of stability training using a large inflatable rubber ball).

- Get outside and strength train for more motivation. Work out with a buddy.

- Join a "Hot Iron" or circuit-training class.

- Ask an instructor to help you design a program using resistance machines. Make sure you know how to modify the program as you improve.

I know a little bit about weight training.

- Find a routine that is specific to your sport or physical condition.

- Find a buddy. Set up a routine.

- Get some training as a refresher in technique.

- Experiment with different modes of strength training.

I'm experienced in strength training and have been doing it for years.

- Get out of the gym and try something new in which you can use your body strength. For example, take up rock climbing, kayaking, or downhill skiing. Identify your weak spots and work on these.

- Try a course in alternative or functional weight training, such as Swiss ball, Pilates, or power yoga.

- Redesign your strength program and learn alternative exercises using free weights.

Flexibility Training

Bend. Twist. Flex. Stretch. Reach. All these movements create a greater range of motion, which gives us more energy in our life. Flexibility training increases range of motion, the ability to move joints freely and completely. Everyone needs range of motion to complete daily tasks. By stretching, muscles lengthen and become more relaxed. By not stretching, muscles become shorter and tighter. Without regular stretching, your range of motion or elasticity becomes retarded and impairs your ability to function fully in all your activities.

As you might guess, a person's need for flexibility differs from every other person's. For example, certain athletic performers such as gymnasts, swimmers, and springboard divers need tremendous flexibility to perform well in their events. The average individual doesn't need that level of flexibility. Nevertheless, everyone needs an unrestricted range of motion in order to meet the day-to-day demands of reaching for a book, bending over to pick up a toy, or getting dressed.

Flexibility depends on muscle elasticity, which, in turn, determines the distance you can lengthen a muscle or rotate a joint. Regular flexibility exercises result in greater agility and speed and, most important, less of a chance that you might injure muscles, tendons, and ligaments. Typically, elasticity decreases with age, but if you stretch regularly, you will lose little, if any.

Make stretching a regular part of your day. If you do, you'll retain great range of motion for the rest of your life. If you don't, you'll someday join the ranks of those who can no longer play sports, reach over to tie their shoes, or bend to talk to a grandchild.

To stay on track with a regular flexibility program, you must manage your time well. Set aside a part of your physical training time for flexibility work, committing yourself to at least 3 to 5 times per week for 10 to 20 minutes for static or contract/relax stretching (more about that later). You might also do it first thing in the morning every morning or for 15 minutes any time of day, at home or in the gym. You have no excuse not to stretch because it requires no special equipment or apparel and can be performed almost anywhere.

Have fun when you stretch by listening to music, stretching with a friend or partner, or stretching during some of your television-watching time. Set some stretching goals and challenges for yourself. If you like keeping records, add flexibility activities and times to your personal fitness log.

Designing a Stretching Program

Stretching your body is important to maintain your range of motion. To develop a daily routine, start with 1 session of 5 to 20 minutes per week, adding 1 each week for 5 to 7 weeks until you're doing it 5 to 7 times per week. Or progress to 10 to 30 minutes per workout 2 to 5 times per week. Your stretching time should increase as you hold each stretch for longer periods of time. For example, in the first few weeks, hold each stretching position for 10 seconds, with 1 repetition. As you progress, hold the stretch or position for longer, increasing the number of repetitions each week by one until you reach four repetitions of each stretch.

How hard should you stretch? It all depends. But, as a rule, you should lengthen a muscle until it feels slightly uncomfortable and hold it at that point for 10 to 20 seconds. The intensity or discomfort level of the stretch goes up when you add to the distance you lengthen the muscle or increase its range of motion.

There are 9 different primary stretches, which include all of the major muscle groups. The following stretching table shows a sample program for stretching that relies on the 9 major stretches. Diagrams of how to perform each stretch follow.

The Fit *and* Fat Stretching Plan

Week	Periodization	Duration of Each Stretch	Number of Repeats	Frequency (Times per Week)
1	Start	10 to 15 seconds	1	1
2	Easy progression	15 to 20 seconds	2	2
3	Easy progression	20 to 25 seconds	2	2
4	Easy progression	20 to 30 seconds	3	3
5	Easy progression	25 to 30 seconds	3	3 to 4
6	Maintenance	30 seconds	4	3 to 5

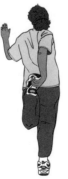

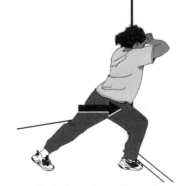

Front, upper leg, quadricep stretch.   *Back, lower leg, calf stretch.*

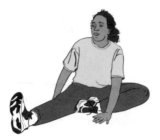

Back, upper leg, hamstring stretch.

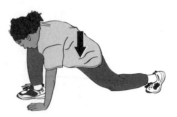

Lower back, hip, and groin stretch.

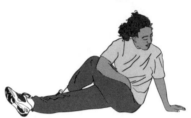

Hip and back stretch.

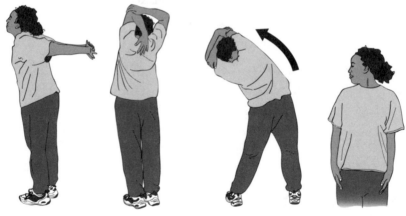

Shoulder stretch.   Tricep stretch.   Side stretch.   Neck stretch.

Follow these simple guidelines when you are stretching, to ensure a safe workout:

- Always breathe fully as you stretch and between stretches.
- Do not bounce while stretching: You will activate a contraction response within the muscles.

- Try to keep the joints (especially the knee, neck, and back) slightly in a bent position, not in full or complete extension.
- Do not stretch to the point that you stress the joint or the muscle. Be gentle.
- Do not stretch until you feel pain.
- Avoid overextension or flexion of the spine.

In addition to structured stretching, participating in certain health and wellness activities will further help you increase your flexibility and range of motion. Try them. They're fun:

- Yoga
- Pilates
- Horseback riding
- Rock climbing
- Ballet dancing
- Gymnastics
- Martial arts

Activity 6.5: Stretching for Life

Write a list of the stretches that you plan to do as part of your flexibility program, making sure you know how to execute each one safely and effectively. Tack pictures of them on the wall in the area where you stretch. Write when you plan to do them in your personal fitness log. Some of the time you allocate can be incorporated into playing with your children or spending time with friends. Add time, too, to the beginning and end of other strength training or cardiovascular training workouts so you can stretch. When you can, add stretching to talking to friends or waiting in a line.

Week 5 Summary

This week, you found out a lot about the value of a sound mind in a sound body. Adding to the metabolic fitness training you learned about last week and the energy black box you discovered in week 3, you are now learning all the skills you need for your Fit *and* Fat Personal Activity Program. I'm really excited for you—you've already made so many changes in your life. Congratulations! You're well along on your journey to becoming an athlete.

We still have a way to go, but don't worry about that for now. Relish your progress. Affirm your commitment. Build on your solid foundation for success: an awareness of your physical and biochemical uniqueness, and a knowledge of how to find the best metabolic, emotional, and physical fitness training for you. In the next chapter, I talk more about fat burning. Then in week 7 it's time to set up some individual goals to focus your training, build your own training program, and put it into practice. Finally, in week 8, you'll learn some skills to help you get back on the wagon if you fall off, and you'll learn ways to keep motivated.

CHAPTER 7

Week 6: Fat Burning

Lighting the Fire Within

Fat burning is a hot subject, particularly if you are concerned about your fatness. Maybe you believe that the one and only goal of any exercise program for you would be fat burning, or maybe you have heard that there is a magic training zone called the "Fat-Burning Zone." Perhaps you are curious how you've managed to get this far into a book on fitness and fatness and dealing with heart zones and emotional zones but have not yet encountered the fat-burning zone? Well, I'd like to tell you right now, right up front, that there is no magic about fat burning. There are, however, a lot of myths. What I'd like to do is to set the record straight for you once and for all with the information in this chapter. I want you to understand not only the myths of fat burning but also the magic of fat burning as part of a program that focuses on metabolic, emotional, and physical fitness. Let's start with some of the myths.

Exposing the Fat-Burning Myth: Phillip's Story

Phillip Whalen is a young professional working as a stockbroker in the city of London. After graduating with a good degree at age 23, he went straight to work for a well-known firm of stockbrokers. In the last four years, he settled into the firm and was promoted three times. He bought himself a trendy loft apartment near the Thames and has plenty of spare cash to pursue his number-one love in life: surfing.

Having grown up in Hawaii, he has always loved riding the waves. With his blossoming career and good income, he has seized every opportunity to buy the latest and best equipment and fly to the best surfing locations in the world. Phillip has dark hair and skin that easily tans, a ready smile, and, along with a slightly round face, the radiant glow of someone who revels in the outdoor life. Now, however, after four years of the high life that comes with his job, his round face matches a very round belly. He's fat.

One evening, a potential girlfriend made a sly comment about Phillip's resemblance to a Sumo wrestler. Although she meant it jokingly, it stung

Phillip and prompted him to do something about the growing bulge. His closet contained four different sizes of pants; he could wear none but the largest. He decided to try what the other young professionals he knew had already done: join a health club and get a personal trainer.

A colleague recommended a personal trainer named Troy. Troy sounded full of enthusiasm on the phone and said he also loved to surf but hadn't done so in years. Troy suggested an initial meeting to assess Phillip's level of fitness, discuss Phillip's goals, and agree on a plan for what they would do together.

Phillip met Troy at the exclusive health club Phillip had joined: huge and fluffy towels, a reception area adorned with Asian orchids, and changing rooms fitted out in green frosted glass and natural rock. Troy led Phillip to the fitness assessment room, where they proceeded to work through the usual health questionnaire, history of medical conditions and illnesses, measurement of height and weight, and skin-fold measurements to determine body fat, all the while maintaining a running conversation about surfing. After Troy did a few quick calculations and filled in a standard results sheet, he offered Phillip his prognosis.

According to Troy, Phillip was 70 pounds over the ideal weight for his height. The skin-fold calipers had given a reading of 35 percent fat, above the 18 percent recommended for a male his age. Troy had calculated that if Phillip could get down to 200 pounds and reduce his body fat percentage to 25 percent, he'd both look and feel better. He wouldn't be rail-thin, but he would certainly be healthier.

So what should Phillip do? He should, Troy recommended, adopt a fat-burning program. What does that involve? Long workouts at a low intensity. Why? Because at low-intensity exercise, the body burns more fat as a percentage of the calories burned than at higher intensities. Troy explained that at high intensities, the body burns only sugar, not body fat. This amazed Phillip, who had assumed that the harder you go, the more fat you burned. But it also made his goal of reaching 200 pounds seem much more reachable.

Phillip immediately began what Troy called the "Slow Burn Fast" program. The first eight weeks would focus on fat burning, and only later would Phillip start doing some weight training and other types of training. First, Phillip would train 5 times a week, at a heart rate of between 60 and 70 percent of maximum heart rate. He was to spend 20 minutes each on a treadmill, a rower, and a stationary cycle, which he would use alternately in order to add variety to his workouts.

Troy also gave Phillip information about healthful eating that convinced him to cut down on the quick fast-food meals he grabbed for lunch. And they agreed to measure Phillip's progress weekly for two months.

Does any of this sound familiar?

If you are fat and you've ever consulted a fitness professional about fat loss, you've probably heard that you should focus on the fat-burning zone, that elusive place where you burn the most calories. It's hard to know when you reach this magic fat-burning zone, but when you do get there and stay there long enough, the fat miraculously burns away, leaving you looking and feeling better. That's such attractive advice. Sadly, however, it's dead wrong.

Dr. Carl Foster, Ph.D., a professor at the Human Performance Laboratory at the University of Wisconsin–La Crosse, argues that the concept of the fat-burning zone was actually one of the most damaging contributions of the fitness industry to people's health and fitness. In reality, there is no such thing as a standard range of heart rates (for example 60 to 70 percent) at which we all burn the most fat—and, contrary to conventional wisdom, focusing on fat burning is *not* the most effective way to lose fat. In this chapter, I show you …

- Why fat-burning programs can keep a person fat and make a fit person unfit.
- Why fit people burn more fat.
- That the fat-burning zone is a myth.
- Why optimum fat burning occurs in a range of heart rates, not just one.
- The value of max fat burning.
- How to enlarge your fat-burning range.

First of all, I explain how the body burns fat and why it is such an important fuel for us. Then I discuss what happens to our fat-burning capacity if we are unconditioned and how it changes when we participate in physical training. Then you'll understand why the fat-burning zone is a myth, that fat burning occurs over a range of heart beats that is unique to each individual. I give you a method for finding your fat-burning range and improving your fat-burning potential, and I recommend a range of workouts that focus on your fitness levels while enhancing your fat-burning results.

The Fire Inside

The body uses two forms of fuel: fat and carbohydrate. It can also use protein, but protein plays such a minor role that we'll omit it from this discussion. The carbohydrate functions like dry kindling: It burns fast, and you can't get going without it. Fat is like coal: It provides most of the energy for the fire and creates long-lasting embers. The body likes to store fat whenever it can. Even the bodies of lean adults store more than 100,000 calories of fat, 50 times the amount of carbohydrate it stores. But, just like a fire that can't get by on just kindling or coal, your body needs to burn a mixture of carbohydrate and fat.

How much energy have you tucked away in your fat stores? How far could your fat stores take you if you accessed it all? When I first met Lorraine, she amused me in a Heart Zones seminar by calculating that she could theoretically run a total of 35 marathons nonstop based on the calories stored in her excess body fat. Here's what she showed me:

1. Current weight in pounds: 202 pounds

2. Percentage of body fat: 44 percent

3. Percentage of excess body fat (total current level — recommended level): 19 percent

4. Number of pounds of excess fat (total body weight × percentage that is excess body fat): 38 pounds

5. Number of calories in excess body fat (3,500 calories × number of pounds): 133,000 calories

6. Number of calories used per hour jogging at 6 miles per hour (4.2 calories × body weight in pounds): 849 calories

7. Number of calories used for one marathon (calories for one marathon × 4.5): 3,820 calories

8. Number of marathons Lorraine could run on excess fat stores: 133,000 ÷ 3,820 = 35

Of course, the body cannot function on fat alone. It always needs some carbohydrate to keep it going, too. And it's obviously impossible for a person to run 35 marathons without stopping and recovering. However, you might find it interesting to apply Lorraine's calculation to yourself. Use the following form to help you.

Activity 7.1: How Far Could Your Fat Take You?

1. Current weight in pounds: _____ pounds

2. Percentage body fat: _____ percent

3. Percentage of excess body fat (total current level — minimum recommended level from the following table): ____ percent − ____ percent (from table) = ____ percent

Recommended Levels of Body Fat

Age	Males	Females
10 to 30	10 to 18 percent	20 to 25 percent
31 to 40	13 to 19 percent	21 to 27 percent
41 to 50	14 to 20 percent	22 to 28 percent
51 to 60	16 to 20 percent	22 to 30 percent
60+	17 to 21 percent	22 to 31 percent

4. Number of pounds of excess body fat (total body weight × percentage that is excess body fat): body weight _____ pounds × _____ percent excess body fat = _____ pounds excess body fat

5. Number of calories in excess body fat: (3,500 calories × number of pounds of spare body fat): 3,500 calories × _____ pounds spare fat = _____ calories

6. Number of calories used per hour jogging at 6 miles per hour: (4.2 calories × body weight in pounds): 4.2 calories × body weight _____ pounds = _____ calories/hour

7. Number of calories used for one marathon: (calories per hour *multiplied* by 4.5): _____ calories/hour [from 6 above]) × 4.5 = _____ calories for one marathon

8. Number of marathons I could run on spare fat stores: (number of calories in spare fat store *divided* by number of calories for one marathon): calories in fat store _____ calories (from 5 above) ÷ calories for one marathon _____ (from 7 above) = _____ number of marathons

Let's take a look at how the body uses fat and carbohydrate. Its carbohydrate is present in the form of blood glucose stored in the liver and the muscles. A 150-pound man's body might contain these carbohydrate resources:

Muscle glycogen	1,400 calories
Liver glycogen	320 calories
Blood glucose	80 calories
Total	1,800 calories

The body can break down its glucose into energy quite quickly. It's the fast fuel you use when you first start to exercise, the fuel the body grabs first in an emergency or stressful situation. The brain cannot function without a constant supply of glucose. That's why diabetics with low blood sugar can go into a coma: The body shuts down all unnecessary functions to survive. To a lesser extent, the same things happens to runners or other endurance athletes who get the "bonk," or "hit the wall," or are caught by the "man with the hammer." When you "bonk," you suddenly feel overwhelmed by a feeling of tiredness. Your blood glucose level has plummeted because it's been nearly all used up by the exercise, and your body responds by telling you to stop.

The body breaks down the fat you eat into fatty acids, which it stores by adding glycerol to make triglycerides. There are plasma triglycerides in the blood, and stores kept in the intramuscular triglycerides in the muscles, and adipose tissue in special fat cells called adipocytes.

Just like a campfire, the burning of both carbohydrate and fat requires oxygen and results in waste products, including carbon dioxide. This type of burning takes place inside special structures within the cells called mitochondria, so-called powerhouses of the body. They contain all the enzymes and chemical structures required for burning carbohydrate and fat as fuel. The mitochondria need oxygen to do their job, and they get it from the blood that flows to the muscles.

However, while you can put out a fire by removing its oxygen supply, your body can keep on burning fuel even when the oxygen supply is limited. As exercise intensity increases, you reach a point at which the oxygen demand from metabolism exceeds the oxygen that the lungs and heart can deliver. When that happens, the mitochondria cannot maintain the normal processes of burning of carbohydrate and fat, so at this point, another type of metabolism kicks in. Anaerobic metabolism burns carbohydrate exclusively, an already limited energy source. Disastrously, however, the waste products of anaerobic metabolism gradually turn off the aerobic metabolism (fat and carbohydrate burning with oxygen) until you are burning pure carbohydrate. Burning up carbohydrate in anaerobic exercise can be sustained for only a matter of minutes, during which you feel the "burn," as a waste product called lactate builds up in the muscles and soon forces you to stop.

How your body balances its fuel use between carbohydrate and fat, both at rest and during physical activity, plays an incredibly significant role in our fitness and our fatness. Good fat burners can train harder and longer before they run out of steam. Good fat burners can burn up the fat they eat and not gain weight so easily. Poor fat burners, on the other hand, get tired easily as their bodies burn up carbohydrate, and they gain weight as their bodies store up the fat.

When you run low on carbohydrate, your body tells you to eat something. Quite likely you will eat a mixture of carbohydrates and fats (as well as protein) in your meal, but your body puts the fat to one side and assigns just the carbohydrates for fuel. In this scenario, it's easy to keep on gaining more and more fat. But I have good news for you! Fitness gives you a means to *change* your fat-burning metabolism for the better. Becoming a better fat burner will lower your propensity for increasing your body fat, and it will improve your endurance for not only fitness training, but all aspects of your life.

Using Fuels During Exercise

Bear with me, please, because this gets a bit complicated. Scientists call it "substrate metabolism," and even they admit that they don't fully understand it. We do know the basics, though. As a rule, the harder you exercise, the more the body relies on carbohydrates as a fuel. Also, the harder you train, the more you increase your rate of fat burning, *up to a certain point of individual maximum fat burning.* After that point, fat burning plummets until you're burning pure carbohydrate.

What does this mean to you and your fitness program? It means you should bear in mind three simple fat-burning rules:

1. As exercise intensity increases, the proportion of fat as a percentage of the total calories burned decreases (see the following figure).

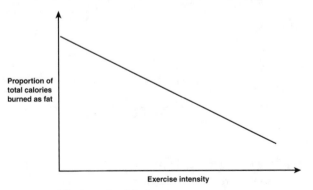

The first rule of fat burning.

2. As exercise intensity increases, so does fat burning (see the following figure).

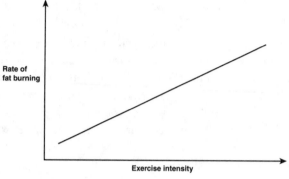

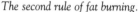

The second rule of fat burning.

3. Fat can burn only in the presence of oxygen.

Combined, rules 2 and 3 mean that exercise increases fat burning up to a maximum point. At this point, when the demand for oxygen from aerobic metabolism exceeds the rate of supply, fat burning starts to plummet (see the following figure). After the body reaches the point of maximum fat burning, it enters the realm of anaerobic carbohydrate metabolism, which causes a rapid buildup in the waste product lactate that inhibits fat-burning metabolism and tells you to stop.

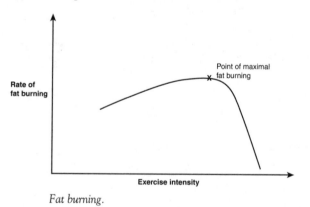

Fat burning.

All this explains how our fuel-burning system shifts as we train harder. Look at the following figure, which shows the relative contribution of fat and carbohydrate to energy burned as exercise intensity increases through the five heart zones. In Zone 1, fat accounts for most of the calories burned, with only a small amount coming from carbohydrate. In Zone 2, you burn more fat, but a smaller ratio of fat to carbohydrate. This trend continues in Zone 3, where more fat but even more carbohydrate is burned. In Zone 4, something interesting starts to happen. Compared to Zone 3, more fat is burned, but a huge amount more of carbohydrate is burned. But at the top of Zone 4, the increase stops and fat burning actually starts to decrease. In Zone 5, hardly any fat is burned, but carbohydrate is burning like a forest fire.

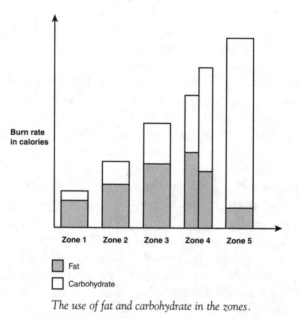

The use of fat and carbohydrate in the zones.

What happened in Zone 4? Well, think back to our three rules of fat burning. Somewhere in Zone 4, the body failed to meet the mitochondria's demand for oxygen. Without additional oxygen, the mitochondria could not increase their rate of fat burning any further, so anaerobic metabolism of carbohydrate kicked in to get the energy needed to up the intensity. Thus began the inhibition of the work of the mitochondria. Up in Zone 5, the energy demand continued to rise, but only the anaerobic metabolism could supply the necessary energy. More anaerobic metabolism meant more inhibition of fat burning and more consumption of carbohydrate.

Influencing Your Fat-Burning Ability

The body's regulation of fat burning is extremely complicated. It involves coordination of the nervous system, the hormones, and the circulatory system to get adipocytes to give up their stored fat and to get blood flow to adipose tissue and working muscles. A healthy body needs the right balance of hormones and enzymes, and the right amount of blood flow to the right organs, fat deposits, and muscles all at the right time. All aspects of your fat burning depend on optimum metabolic, emotional, and physical fitness.

Hormones figure prominently in the regulation of fat burning, and not just the sex hormones, although progesterone, estrogen, and testosterone can greatly influence fat burning. Actually, insulin is the single most important hormone in the regulation of fat burning because it helps control blood glucose levels. When we eat a meal, the carbohydrates are converted, some quickly and others more slowly, to glucose, which enters the bloodstream. Whenever glucose gets too high, the pancreas quickly releases insulin. Insulin tells the cells to grab the glucose quickly, either to use right away or to store it. This prevents the glucose levels from getting dangerously high, and it provides stores of carbohydrate that the body can use later. But in addition to telling the body what to do with glucose, insulin tells the cells of the body what to do with fat: High insulin levels send the message to stop burning fat. Even a tiny increase in insulin levels can suppress fat burning to very low levels.

Insulin works antagonistically with other hormones called the catecholamines. These include norepinephrine and epinephrine. Whereas insulin tells fat cells to hold on to their fat, these other hormones tell the fat cells to release their fat into the bloodstream. When we start to exercise, insulin levels fall and catecholamine levels rise, causing the adipocytes, or fat cells, to release their fat into the bloodstream.

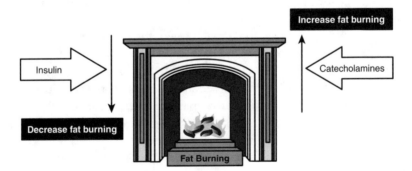

Hormonal regulation of fat burning.

Fitness training improves the actions of the fat-burning hormones. As we saw in Chapter 5, when we explored metabolic fitness, the cells become more sensitive to insulin during training. As you become fitter, the cells become more sensitive to the catecholamine hormones, too.[1] As you get fitter, the adipocytes or fat cells need to get only a whiff of the catecholamine hormones to know it's time to start releasing fat into the bloodstream. In addition to the specialized fat stores, the body stores fat close to where it will use it: as intramuscular triglycerides. The regulation of fat release from these stores is carried out by a hormone called triglyceride lipase. Exercise increases the amount of fat stored as intramuscular triglycerides. This is good news because after exercise, the body puts the fat you eat in the intramuscular triglycerides instead of the fat depots (your hips and bottom). Exercise increases the levels of triglyceride lipase and makes its action more efficient.[2] Low- to moderate-intensity training best delivers this benefit.

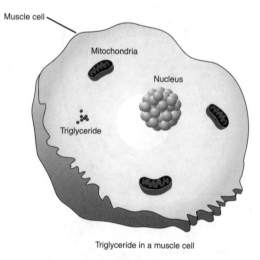

Triglyceride in a muscle cell

Intramuscular triglycerides.

Enzymes and other chemical structures, such as transport proteins that truck fat around the body, play a vital role, too. Note the trucks in the following figure. Fat cells and muscle cells maintain docking stations made up of transport proteins where materials can enter or exit the cell. The docking stations function like porches where the transport proteins can load and unload their fat. The body makes only the quantity of trucks and docking stations it needs. Fitness training stimulates the body to make more trucks and more docking stations.[3] The more trucks and docking stations there are, the more efficiently the materials, including fat, can move from point to point. As the body gets more fit, the muscles get more docking stations for accepting fat in the cell, and the mitochondria, the powerhouses within the muscle cells, get more docking stations to accept the fat they need. The whole fat-transport system becomes more efficient.[4] Again, low to moderate exercise intensities appear to be the best stimulus for these kinds of fat-burning improvements.

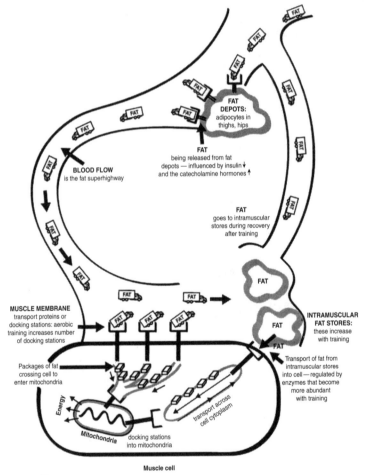

Fat transport.

Mitochondria, the powerhouses of the cells, are enclosed structures within the cells. Full of enzymes, they are constantly buzzing with chemical reactions. As the body asks the cells to do more work, the mitochondria multiply and grow bigger. Obviously, if you want to burn fuel faster, more and larger power generators will help you do that.

Circulation also helps regulate fuel burning, particularly fat burning. The circulation system functions like a superhighway for fat, transporting it to where it's needed. During exercise, blood flow to the adipose tissues can double, while flow to the muscles can increase by as much as 25 times.[5] Remember the third rule of fat burning? Fat burns only in the presence of oxygen. Because fat burns only inside the mitochondria, the efficiency of the circulatory system in delivering oxygen is crucial to fat burning. Once the demand for oxygen exceeds the supply, anaerobic metabolism kicks in, inhibiting fat burning. The body can delay the onset of anaerobic metabolism by more efficiently getting oxygen to the mitochondria. It does this by improving the network of capillaries to the muscle cells, strengthening and enlarging the heart muscle so that it can pump more blood with each heartbeat, and creating more hemoglobin to carry the oxygen. When the body becomes more efficient at delivering oxygen, the point at which increased oxygen demand exceeds oxygen supply is raised. Now you can exercise harder before anaerobic metabolism reduces your fat burning. In contrast to hormone and enzyme changes, these changes occur at moderate to intense levels of exercise that challenge the cardiorespiratory system.

Take a look at the following figure. This represents the fat transport of a fit person. It shows more trucks and more docking stations and a wider fat superhighway. A traffic cop directs the fat trucks directly to the intramuscular fat stores, thereby reducing the number of fat deliveries to the fat depots. Note the increased number and size of the mitochondria and the quicker transport of fat across the cell to the mitochondria.

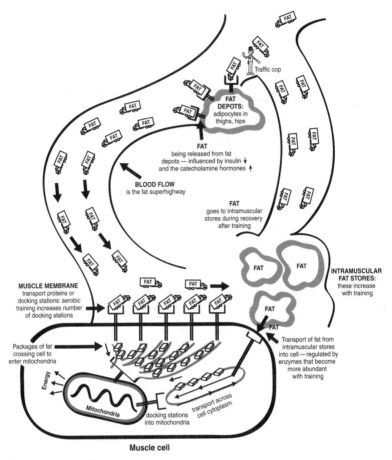

Fat transport in a fit person.

Expanding Your Fat-Burning Potential

You probably suspect from the previous discussion of fat burning that you can expand your potential for fat burning by becoming fitter. Changes caused by fitness training enhance blood flow. A greater capacity to supply oxygen to the cells, increased sensitivity to fat-burning hormones, and improved levels of fatburning enzymes all make you a better fat burner. Fitness opens the doors to our fat stores. Take another look at the preceding figure showing the use of fat and carbohydrates in the zones, and think about what happens to this fuel-burning pattern as our fitness improves. Then study the following figure.

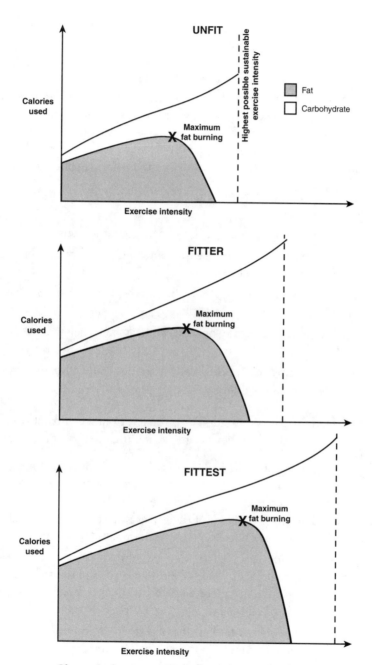

Changes in the pattern of fat and carbohydrate use with improvements in fitness.

Although the actual fat-burning curve differs for each individual, the graph does show you the general direction of the changes that occur when we do fitness training. Notice that the fat-burning curve moves up and to the right as we get fitter. Also note the mix of fuels burned at, say, 70 percent of maximum heart rate. In the conditioned state, the body burns far more calories than an unconditioned person would at the same relative exercise intensity. In addition, a greater proportion of the total calories burned is fat rather than carbohydrate. If you want to open the doors to your fat store, all you need to do is get fitter and fitter. Consider all the amazing benefits of fitness:

- You will be able to exercise harder (walk or run faster) at a given heart rate.
- You will burn more calories per minute at a given exercise intensity.
- At a given relative exercise intensity and heart rate, you will burn a higher proportion of calories as fat.
- You will be able to exercise at a higher intensity and heart rate before you reach your anaerobic threshold.
- You will be able to exercise longer at all heart rates below your anaerobic threshold.
- At rest and during your normal daily activities, you will burn a greater proportion of calories as fat.

Isn't this fantastic news? But don't just take it from me. Take it from the researchers and scientists who have been solving the mystery of fat burning:

- Researchers compared the fuel use of a group of endurance-trained cyclists to a group of untrained volunteers training in Zone 3 for an hour. At one hour, they measured the fuel use. While the untrained men were burning 33 percent of their energy from fat, the trained men were burning 53 percent of their energy from fat.[6]
- A group of previously sedentary women had their fat burning assessed before they trained for 12 weeks. Researchers then reassessed them while they cycled on an indoor bike for one hour in Zone 3. Their fat burning had risen 117 percent after the 12 weeks of training.[7]
- Researchers assessed the fat burning of a group of untrained men at rest before they trained on an indoor cycle for 31 days. After the training, their fat burning during exercise had increased 58 percent and their fat burning at rest had increased by 11 percent. They also exhibited a

100 percent increased dependence on intramuscular triglycerides, a 30 percent lower depletion of glucose from their blood, and a significantly lower lactate accumulation rate.[8]

- In one study, a group of obese men trained for 12 weeks at 60 percent of their maximum heart rate and increased their fat oxidation during low-intensity exercise by 40 percent after a 12-week training program.[9]

- A study examined a group of lean, healthy, sedentary men who trained at 60 percent of their maximum heart rate 3 times a week for 12 weeks. Fat oxidation during exercise was increased by 30 percent after the training, and the men also demonstrated increased levels of fat metabolism enzymes.[10]

Benefiting from Maximal Fat Burning

The preceding figure reveals that fat burning increases to a certain point and then drops off sharply. Researchers call this the point of maximal fat burning, or Fat_{max}.[11] It's a moving point, of course, because the point at which anaerobic metabolism starts to inhibit fat metabolism (the anaerobic threshold) changes with fitness. Thus, the idea of a fixed "fat-burning zone" is ridiculous: Nobody burns fat in the same way, and everybody has his or her own max fat burning point based on their current level of fitness. Your fat burning increases steadily as you exercise, until it reaches maximal fat burning. You improve your fat-burning capacity by training inside your fat-burning range, and you expand it by pushing your max fat burning point higher.

Your individual max fat burning point depends somewhat on your genetics, your level of training in a particular sport, your diet, and what you ate for your last meal and when you ate it. However, the overriding important factor is your level of fitness: Greater fitness equals a higher max fat burning point and a more expansive fat-burning range. In a recent study, researchers who tested 11 moderately trained male cyclists to determine their max fat burning point found enormous variations in their individual results.[12] The lowest max fat burning point occurred at 54 percent of the maximum heart rate, and the highest occurred at 92 percent of the maximum heart rate. For somebody with a maximum heart rate of 180, this corresponds to a variation between 97 bpm and 166 bpm.

The researchers also determined the point after which a cyclist's metabolism completely switches over to carbohydrates, which occurs as exercise intensity increases beyond max fat burning. In just these 11 cyclists, the results ranged from 84 to 98 percent of the maximum heart rate, corresponding to heart rates of 151 bpm and 176 bpm for a person with a maximum heart rate of 180.

In another study using 32 obese subjects with a BMI over 30, scientists found that their anaerobic thresholds, which is a point equating roughly to the max fat burning point, occurred at around 78 percent ± 6 percent of the maximum heart rate.[13] Thus, for a person with a maximum heart rate of 180, the anaerobic threshold could fall anywhere between 130 bpm and 150 bpm. You can see from the variations in the results how important it is to find your own unique max fat burning point. Never rely on a formula or an average to calculate it.

Activity 7.2: Determining Your Max Fat Burning Point

Your anaerobic threshold equates to your point of maximal fat burning, and you can use any number of tests to measure it. You could even have it measured scientifically in a sports laboratory. However, if you learn to listen to the right signals from your body, you'll soon be able to pinpoint your anaerobic threshold, or point of maximal fat burning, without a special test. Listen to your heart, and you will begin to understand its language.

The feeling that signals your anaerobic threshold is the feeling that you can't possibly increase your heart rate by five more beats and sustain it for a period of time. It's the highest heart rate you can maintain for a sustained period. Imagine hiking up a steep hill. What pace can you sustain for the entire climb? While a child or an inexperienced hiker might rush ahead, get tired, and have to stop and rest, someone who has climbed lots of hills before will know how to pace themselves, establishing a rhythm when their heart rate settles at a steady number. A faster rhythm and pace would tire them and force them to stop and catch their breath; they would then have passed their anaerobic threshold. Lorraine describes it this way:

> To me, the feeling of being at my anaerobic threshold is like when you are cycling in a pack of cyclists who are too fast for you. You know when it's too fast because you start to look at your heart rate monitor all the time instead of at the scenery or riders around you. My anaerobic threshold is the number where I feel, "If these guys go any faster, I can't go with them, and I'm going to get dropped from this group."

You can also get a feeling for your anaerobic threshold by taking the talk test. Do it on a piece of indoor exercise equipment such as a cycle or treadmill with a friend or partner. Warm up for 10 minutes to a heart rate of 110 bpm. Now recite the Pledge of Allegiance or the words to a favorite song. Instruct your partner to listen continually as you talk at that exercise intensity. Now increase your heart rate by 10 beats every 2 minutes. At each 2-minute mark, when your heart rate reaches 120, 130, 140, and so on, recite the Pledge. It should get harder and harder to speak clearly. When you can no longer talk comfortably, you have reached your max fat burning point. If you continue to increase your exercise intensity, your anaerobic metabolism will start to kick in and your fat-burning rate will plunge. Note your heart rate number, and gradually bring it back to below 100 over 10 minutes. Your max fat burning point was the heart rate at which you changed from being able to say the Pledge comfortably to being unable to say it without gasping for air.

Training to Enlarge Your Fat-Burning Range

To enlarge your fat-burning range, you need to accomplish two things. First, you need to become a more efficient fat burner by improving your levels of hormones and enzymes. You do this with "metabolic training," or low- to moderate-intensity training. Second, you need to enlarge your fat-burning capacity by increasing your oxygen-delivery capacity, building more mito-chondria, and pushing up your max fat burning point with physical training. These changes are stimulated by moderate- to high-intensity training, or fitness training.

Objective 1: Metabolic Training: Teaching Your Metabolism to Burn Fat

To train your metabolism to burn fat, you must establish new enzyme levels and new levels of fat-burning hormones. You must adjust the way the body stores fat. To achieve this, you should exercise for a long period of time at an exercise intensity at which you are burning a high proportion of fat. This low- to moderate-intensity training should occur at 20 beats or more below your max fat burning point. Training at this level allows your body to adapt com-fortably to the new challenge. The longer the session in metabolic training, the more benefits you'll get. Two examples of metabolic fitness workouts are given in activities 7.3 and 7.4.

Objective 2: Fitness Training: Raising Your Anaerobic Threshold

You can effectively raise your anaerobic threshold by training "at-about-and-around" your anaerobic threshold, or at 5 to 10 beats on either side of your numerical anaerobic threshold number. For example, Lorraine's anaerobic threshold for running is 146. Therefore, an anaerobic threshold workout for Lorraine would be in the range of 136 to 156 heartbeats.

Interval training raises your anaerobic threshold especially well. For instance, train for a series of 2-minute intervals, working out at an intensity 15 to 20 beats above your anaerobic threshold for 2 minutes and then recovering at well below your anaerobic threshold for 2 minutes. It's hard training, so take special care not to injure yourself. Work up to it gradually over weeks or even months. An example of such a physical fitness training workout is given in Activity 7.5.

Balancing Your Act

Physical fitness training and metabolic fitness training deliver two different benefits. With physical fitness training, you teach your body to become fitter—the heart becomes stronger; with metabolic training, you stimulate your body to make biochemical adaptations. But you need both because neither will work without the other. If you focus on only metabolism training (at low intensity), you won't get the benefit of getting fitter and boosting your fat-burning rates over a wider range of heart rates. If you focus only on fitness training (at high intensity), you may not give your body a chance to put its chemical house in order and help you get the fat out and the energy where you need it. To build a weekly program around fat burning ...

- Do at least one interval session per week that includes a brief time above your max fat burning point.
- Every week include one or two training sessions "at-about-and-around" your max fat burning point.

Burning Fat While Working Out

Here are some examples of key workouts you can use as part of a fat-burning workout. The first two provide metabolic training; the third physical fitness training workout helps you push up your max fat burning point by building a bigger engine.

Activity 7.3: Talking Off the Fat

This workout keeps you in the metabolic fitness zones and allows you to catch up on the latest gossip at the same time. You need a partner for this one, preferably somebody who loves to talk. The activity revolves around your talk threshold heart rate (TTHR), a very narrow range of heartbeats perched on the heart rate threshold that allows you to keep talking. Don't confuse this with the talk test you used to find your max fat burning point: That threshold is much higher. Your TTHR is where you can cycle, jog, or dance along while carrying on a conversation comfortably. You want to maintain this heart rate throughout this workout.

Choose an activity that you love, and invite a friend to join you. Any activity in which you get sweaty but not so out of breath that you can't talk will work fine. Spend the first five minutes warming up slowly. Over the next five minutes, gradually increase the intensity until you reach a level at which you can still keep your conversation going but couldn't if you went any faster. It may take a little trial and error to find this point. You're now working out at your TTHR. Settle into enjoying your time with your friend and your activity, whether you are cycling, line dancing, or skating. Over the next 40 minutes, glance at your heart rate monitor to ensure that you remain at your TTHR. Finally, take 10 to 15 minutes to bring your heart rate down gradually by slowing and then stopping your activity.

Activity 7.4: Moving Your Metabolism

For this workout, choose a piece of indoor cardiovascular exercise equipment or do outdoor walking, running, or skating. Actually, any activity in which you can adjust the intensity will work fine. With it you will be training in the lower two heart rate zones and just creeping into Zone 3 for six minutes of your workout.

Review your heart rate numbers before you start, jotting them in the following table so you don't have to think about them as you go along. Then just follow the workout plan. Your heart rate profile would resemble that in the following figure.

Elapsed Time (Min)	Workout Plan	Heart Zone	Your Heart Rate (bpm)	Interval Time (Min)
0 to 3	Warm up in Z1.	1	_____	3
3 to 5	Warm up to the bottom of Z2.	2	_____	2

Activity 7.4. *continued*

Elapsed Time (Min)	Workout Plan	Heart Zone	Your Heart Rate (bpm)	Interval Time (Min)
5 to 29	Increase HR 10 bpm and sustain for 2 minutes. Then increase intensity to bottom of Z3 and sustain for 2 minutes, followed by going back to bottom of Z2 for 2 minutes. Repeat a total of 4 times for a total of 6 minutes in Z3.	2	_____	2
		3	_____	2
		2	_____	2 (× 4 = 24)
32 to 35	Cool down to Z1.	1	_____	3

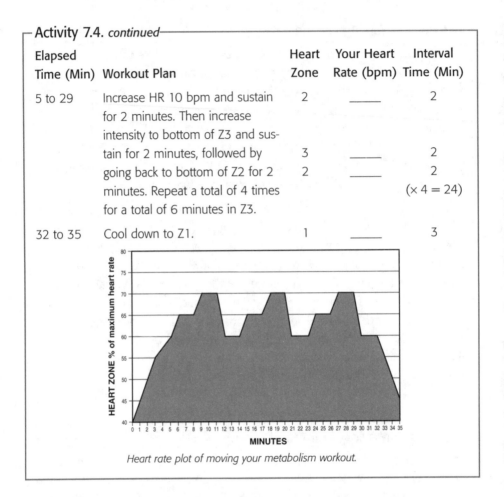

Heart rate plot of moving your metabolism workout.

Activity 7.5: Exercising "At-About-and-Around" Your Max Fat Burning Point

Now we come to a workout that can really challenge you. But there's no better way to push up your anaerobic threshold and max fat burning point. Don't attempt it until you have been training long enough to do it confidently and safely. Make sure you have determined your max fat burning point before you do this workout.

Select any activity that lends itself to a full range of intensity. Write your heart rate numbers on the chart before you start, using your own individual anaerobic threshold number (AT) and the following form. Complete the column showing which zone you will be training in. Your heart rate profile should resemble that in the following figure.

Elapsed Time (Min)	Workout Plan	Heart Zone	Your Heart Rate (bpm)	Interval Time (Min)
0 to 5	Warm up to the bottom of Z2.	2	_____	5
5 to 10	Increase HR to bottom of Z3.	3	_____	5
10 to 12	Increase HR to AT plus 5 bpm.		_____	2
12 to 14	Decrease HR 5 bpm to AT.		_____	2
14 to 16	Increase HR 5 bpm.		_____	2
16 to 18	Decrease HR 5 bpm.		_____	2
18 to 20	Increase HR 5 bpm.		_____	2
20 to 22	Decrease HR 5 bpm.		_____	2
22 to 24	Increase HR 5 bpm.		_____	2
24 to 26	Decrease HR 5 bpm.		_____	2
26 to 28	Increase HR 5 bpm.		_____	2
28 to 30	Decrease HR 5 bpm.		_____	2
30 to 36	Decrease HR to midpoint of Z3.	3	_____	3
36 to 56	Repeat minutes 10 to 30.	Various	_____	20
56 to 58	Decrease HR to bottom of Z3.	3	_____	2
58 to 60	Cool down to bottom of Z2.	2	_____	2

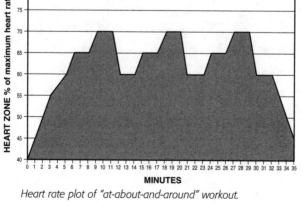

Heart rate plot of "at-about-and-around" workout.

185

Activity 7.6: Feeling the Burn

This workout takes you above your anaerobic threshold. It is the most effective way to raise that threshold and your max fat burning point. During the workout, you will spend a few minutes at a time at a heart rate that you cannot sustain for long. *Caution:* You *must* rest between each interval. This is such a grueling workout; don't attempt it until you have been training long enough to do it safely. If you haven't done this workout before, or if you find 10 intervals too much to handle, start with just 3 or 4 and gradually build up to 10. This workout comes with another warning: Prepare yourself for sore muscles tomorrow!

Pick an activity in which you can alter the intensity quickly and easily. Not all pieces of indoor exercise equipment permit you to increase your heart rate by up to 30 beats a minute over a very short period. Complete the following workout plan table with your heart rate and zone numbers. Your heart rate profile at the end of the workout should resemble the next figure. Keep moving in the rest periods and try to catch your breath. If you experience *any* pain during this workout, aside from the discomfort of hard training, stop immediately.

Elapsed Time (Min)	Workout Plan	Heart Zone	Your Heart Rate (bpm)	Interval Time (Min)
0 to 2	Warm up to midpoint of Z1.	1	_____	2
2 to 7	Warm up to midpoint of Z2.	2	_____	5
7 to 9	Increase HR to bottom of Z3.	2, 3	_____	2
9 to 12	Increase HR to 10 beats above AT, and sustain for 2 minutes.	Depends	_____	3
13	Recover to bottom of Z3.	Depends	_____	1
14 to 29	Repeat this interval four times.	Depends	_____	15
29 to 32	Recover to bottom of Z2, and sustain for two minutes.		_____	3
33	Increase HR to bottom of Z3.	2, 3	_____	1
34 to 36	Increase HR to 10 beats above AT, and sustain for two minutes.	Depends	_____	3

Elapsed Time (Min)	Workout Plan	Heart Zone	Your Heart Rate (bpm)	Interval Time (Min)
37	Recover to bottom of Z3.	Depends	_____	1
38 to 53	Repeat the interval four times.	Depends	_____	15
54 to 60	Cool down to bottom of Z1.	Various	_____	6

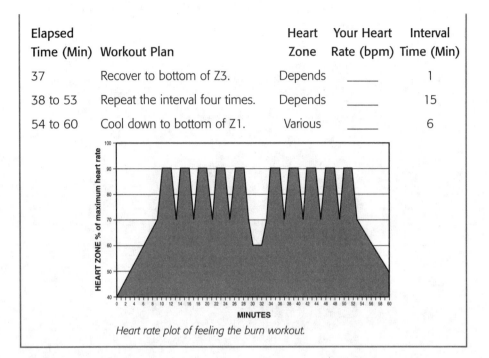

Heart rate plot of feeling the burn workout.

Week 6 Summary

Hopefully, you've learned enough about fat burning in this week that you can incorporate it into your lifelong fitness plan. With your better understanding of how the body burns fuel and balances its use of fat and carbohydrate, you can avoid the trap of following a typical fat-burning program handed out by those in the fitness industry. You now possess the tools to identify your point of maximal fat burning and to train in ways that will enlarge your fat-burning range. Enlarging your fat-burning range will give you access to the body's most precious and largest asset: your fat reserves. When you become a better fat burner, you become a healthier, happier person with a better chance of living a longer, more active life.

CHAPTER 8

Week 7: Tailored to Fit

Building Your Unique Personal Activity Program

Over the last seven weeks of this program, you have learned a lot about fitness and fatness and have made some remarkable discoveries about your own physiology. Up until now, you've been following the suggestions each week for different types of metabolic, emotional, and physical fitness training activities. I've tried to introduce you progressively to each type of training and make the activities flexible enough for anybody to complete. Now it's time to think about going it alone, being your own coach, building your *own* plan. Maybe you've tried to get fit in the past and failed? This time you will succeed: You have many new tools and ideas. But they will only work if you plan what you are going to do.

Planning to Succeed: Kelly's Story

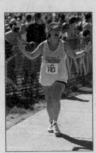

Kelly is a 42-year-old woman with three children who has planned to be fit. She has been a devoted wife and mother for the last 16 years, supporting her husband through several marathons and helping her children accumulate trophies in soccer, basketball, football, swimming, and baseball. However, Kelly herself had never participated in a sporting event. She didn't identify herself as athletic at all. Oh, she had tried getting in shape dozens of times, but each time she'd failed. This time, she vowed, she would train for her first triathlon. After months of dedicated training, she succeeded. Why did she choose something as challenging as a triathlon? What did she do differently "this time"? What influenced her to get fit, and what helped her achieve her goal? After crossing that finish line of the triathlon, she e-mailed me her thoughts about those guidelines:

For several years, I've been trying to get back in shape and have never accomplished the goal. Occasionally, I'd hear someone talk about their experience in the Danskin Triathlon, and I'd think, "I could do that!" I registered online with little thought as to how I would accomplish this feat. Several friends said they would sign up and do the race with me, but they didn't. A few friends even laughed when I told them what I was doing. However, my husband and three children remained supportive!

I attended the race orientation seminar and purchased a Heart Zones training book, training log, and a heart rate monitor. Through the course of the summer, many obstacles kept presenting themselves, including vacations and family demands. I kept persisting and then encountered problems with high blood pressure due to a medication my doctor had prescribed for menstrual problems. Many people tried to persuade me to try the race next year, but I kept moving in the direction of race day. I was so frightened the day before race day, but I attended the registration anyway. I listened to Sally Edwards speak and knew that I had to try. I adopted the race mantra and became a great swimmer, a great biker, and a great runner (well, walker mostly). I tried to believe that Sally truly would be there for me if I were, in fact, the last finisher.

The anxiety of race day is comparable to the anxiety of giving birth. The mass of women and equipment was overwhelming. My legs felt like jelly and my stomach was unstable, but I kept moving forward. I looked across Cherry Creek Reservoir (Denver, Colorado) at the rising sun and was filled with doubt. Then a remarkable moment occurred: My three children wrapped their arms around me and wished me good luck. Somehow my husband had found a way to get them to me before I hit the water. The swim was so scary, but I kept saying my mantra.

At the first red buoy, I was saddened to learn I was only one third of the way to the finish. I kept swimming, and, my God, I finished! I ran to my bike, exhilarated (I loved my bike), and I finished the bike section. I put on my running T-shirt and took off. I had moments of actually jogging that amazed me. I was not last. Incredible! I saw the faces of my family, cameras, people cheering at the finish! Then I hear, "... and Kelly Cantrell from Littleton, Colorado." I was overwhelmed and in shock. My family swarmed around me, and I basked in their pride! I had completed the race in 2 hours, 10 minutes. I am, believe it or not, not just an athlete, but a triathlete.

Kelly, once a mere spectator with no-to-low fitness, became a true athlete when she crossed the finish line of her first triathlon. To get there, she overcame barriers that so many of us face: family responsibilities, a job,

doubts and fears, low self-confidence and body image, no sports back-
ground, and little free personal time. Kelly conquered all those and more.
And she did it because she had set a goal and wouldn't let anything pre-
vent her from reaching her goal. The triathlon event, the exhilaration
of crossing the finish line, motivated her to train for another and then
another event. In fact, her role in life has changed from being a mother
and wife supporting others from the sidelines to being a full participant
in sports and life. None of it happened by accident. It happened because
she discovered what it took to make her plan successful, and Kelly planned
to get fit. In this chapter, you'll build your own unique personal activity
program the same way Kelly did.

Personalizing Your Program

Your unique mind and body deserve an equally unique fitness training plan,
one that provides feedback and motivation tailored to your specific emotional,
physical, and metabolic characteristics. Studies in which researchers trained
all the subjects in exactly the same way found wild variations from individual
to individual. In one study, the benefits ranged from no gain to a doubling in
aerobic fitness.[1] Now researchers recognize that the actual benefits from training depend not so much on age, sex, or ethnic origin as on an individual's current level of fitness.[2] A very fit person can find the "one-size-fits-all" training
too easy and not benefit at all, while a very unfit person could find the same
program too hard. Training bestows huge benefits, but only when the program
matches a person's current position on the fitness continuum.

No program will get results, however, unless you stick to it. Have you
tried to start a program before and found it too hard, too time-consuming, too
uncomfortable, too boring, or just too darned much trouble? Why won't that
happen this time? It will if you don't address the reasons for failure head-on.
By identifying past road blocks, you can factor them into your new program.
Once again, you must confront your own particular set of obstacles, not someone else's.

What else should you consider? Your motivation level, the amount of
external support you receive, your previous experience with sports training,
the demands of your personal life, and your personal goals in life all come
into play. A lot of people drop out because they try to do too much too soon.
Unless you are very fit, you want to start low and go slow. Contrary to the old

cliché, if there's pain, there's no gain. A lot of people also drop out because they don't get enough support and encouragement from family and friends. External support makes a huge difference. That's why group activities such as aerobics or spinning work for so many people.

We live such time-starved lives these days that we find it hard to incorporate *any* new time-consuming activity into our busy schedules. If we do manage to cram it in, we end up with more stress. And nothing kills motivation more than stress. Fortunately, you can overcome all these obstacles if you recognize them and address them when you design your new program. It all starts with a careful and thoughtful self-assessment.

Assessing Yourself

In earlier chapters, you assessed yourself in terms of your emotional, physical, and metabolic fitness. Since your program will take all of that into account, you should pause for a few minutes to review these assessments. Then you can begin to weigh what factors might interfere with your plan and prevent you from going from where you are now to where you want to be in the future.

You don't want to become a fitness drop-out. Statistically, the typical new member of a health club follows a written plan for about three to four weeks before starting to fall off the program. First the person stops going so frequently; then after about six to eight weeks, he or she doesn't go at all. Why? Interrogate a thousand drop-outs, and you'll discover a thousand reasons. Do you know yourself well enough to predict your own reasons *before* you join the ranks of the drop-outs from fitness and a happier, healthier life?

Knocking Out the Drop-Out Bug

Unlike the common cold, there is a cure for the drop-out bug: a healthy dose of knowledge of the truth about fitness and fatness, and knowledge about yourself. Self-knowledge does not come easily—at least, perfectly honest self-knowledge doesn't. How honest can you be with yourself? Making changes in your life and, more important, sticking to those changes requires brutal honesty.

To ensure a maximum level of "sticking power," you need to evaluate your readiness to change, your motivation levels, and other factors such as discomfort while fitness training. Clear and accurate assessment of these elements not only gives you big clues about your own drop-out risk, but it also provides key pointers on the development of your fitness plan that will help you protect yourself against drop-out.

Starting or restarting any sort of program involves a change. Without change, you will not move forward to greater fitness. I know change is not easy for anyone, and that each of us changes our behaviors and our habits in different ways. Fitness training should be a daily health behavior not unlike bathing or brushing your teeth. You know your body requires daily care. Fitness training is daily care, too. Just as it needs vitamins, the body needs a minimum daily requirement of physical activity. Your life depends on it. Your heart craves it. If you aren't doing enough of it, you must make some changes and develop some new habits. And that takes emotional and psychological energy.

Researchers who have studied the emotional and psychological aspects of implementing fitness as a daily habit have discovered that change follows a series of steps. You want to find out your current position in this step-wise progression because that helps determine the components of your unique fitness plan. For example, if you are at the start of the changing process, you'll want to choose activities that will give you instant benefits and a lot of positive reinforcement. They should be fun, comfortable, and socially stimulating. Somebody farther along the changing process might find that setting an athletic goal or getting a training buddy could help him or her stick to the program. Knowing where you are in the process helps you take the next step, and the next, and the next.

Activity 8.1: Preparing to Change

Can you pinpoint your position with respect to the five steps of fitness-training changes? Which description best describes your thinking about your fitness training? Using the following form, check the statements that best describe your approach to fitness, to determine your category of athlete.

The Five Steps of Fitness

Category of athlete you would describe yourself as:

- Step 1: The Spectator
    - ❏ I am not going to start a fitness-training program of any kind.
    - ❏ I don't think there are enough good reasons to get fit.
    - ❏ I don't like fitness training, and I don't get the benefits.
    - ❏ Everyone's trying to get me to work out, but I am not going to do it.

193

Activity 8.1. *continued*

- Step 2: The Speculator
    - ❏ I am just not sure if I want to do a fitness-training program.
    - ❏ I have tried before and always failed.
    - ❏ I think about getting fit, but I don't know if it's worth it.
    - ❏ I don't know if it will work for me right now because there are so many other things going on in my life.

- Step 3: The Sideliner
    - ❏ I know it is time to change, and I need to start soon.
    - ❏ I know I need to get going because the health benefits are important to me.
    - ❏ I am somewhat unsure about whether I can stay on a program.
    - ❏ I know it might be uncomfortable, and I am unsure about whether I am ready for that experience.

- Step 4: The First-Timer
    - ❏ In the last six months, I have started to work out.
    - ❏ I know what I need to do to train, but I'd like to learn more.
    - ❏ I have set some goals for what I would like to gain from my workouts.
    - ❏ Sometimes I get discouraged, but I am confident that if I stick with my plan, it will work.

- Step 5: The Athlete
    - ❏ I fitness-train daily without having to think about it.
    - ❏ I like to train, and I feel confident about it.
    - ❏ I have no reason to quit.
    - ❏ I'd like to do more fitness training.

Each of these five stages represents a different degree of readiness to change. Your fitness-training program should heed your current degree of readiness to change. For example, if you define yourself as a spectator right now and have not committed to making fitness training a daily part of your life, then the program that would help you the most is the one that will get you thinking hard about beginning a program, learning more about the benefits of fitness training, and spending time with friends who work out.

The Five Steps of Fitness Change

This is *not* the time to launch an ambitious, heavy-duty program. You must prepare yourself for that by gradually growing your readiness, by preparing, and by taking each of the five steps that lead you toward thinking of yourself as an athlete. Let's elaborate on each of the steps.

Step 1: The Spectator

You are not thinking about playing. You don't yet see why you should take part in a fitness-training program, and you don't appreciate what you could gain.

Ways to Change

Spectators watch as life goes by and live a life of regrets and "I should haves." Think of someone you love and ask yourself, "Should I start thinking about getting healthier so we can grow old together?" The answer to that question should move you one step toward becoming a speculator. Focus on the benefits of fitness training: reduced risk of cardiovascular disease, increased muscle mass, improved self-esteem, and others. Figure out a way around the roadblocks that are holding you back. Get support from your friends and loved ones. Your program should be fun and easy, requiring no special clothes or equipment. You should involve other people who will help get you motivated.

Activities for Moving Up

Start a walking program. Walking gives you enormous metabolic benefits. There is little to no discomfort. You can walk regardless of the weather (in bad weather, join an indoor program). Walking is one of the very best forms of training because it is inexpensive and something you can do regardless of your current level of fitness. Read more about living a healthful lifestyle, or check out a video from the library, such as Covert Bailey's *Fit or Fat Food and Fitness Foolishness*. Ask a friend to join you for a ballroom dancing class. Dancing is fun, involves listening and moving to music, and gives you a chance to meet new people. As you develop the habit of doing your new physical activity programs such as walking or dancing, you will notice your moods shifting, your mental attitude becoming more positive, and your energy getting stronger.

Step 2: The Speculator

You are seriously thinking about what it will take to fitness train, but you haven't started yet. You understand the benefits but are still thinking about what you would have to give up in order to get these benefits.

Ways to Change

It's time to move from thinking toward doing. The benefits of fitness training far outweigh the costs. Make a list of the real benefits versus the real costs to see the long-term payback. Set some realistic goals, such as reducing stress and feeling better about yourself. Find a role model your age, body type, or whatever is important for you, and see how she or he has benefited from introducing fitness into her or his life. Ask that person what made him or her start and how he or she has managed to stick with the program. Your program shouldn't be overly taxing in terms of intensity, length, or frequency. Start easy.

Activities for Moving Up

You need to find what you love to do. Experiment with activities you think you might enjoy. Try each one time and see what meshes with you, even if you have tried it before. Try swimming, riding a mountain bike, taking a hike in the hills, playing nine holes of golf, sailing a small boat, taking a dog for a walk, or playing games in the park. Try an outdoor adventure activity such as map reading or rafting. Try a game of tennis. Try an aerobics class. Try a martial arts class. Try a piece of home exercise equipment.

Step 3: The Sideliner

You have made the decision to train and are standing on the sideline of the fitness game getting ready to play. Perhaps a friend has challenged you to do an event, or your doctor has insisted that now is the time. You are beginning to promise yourself to take better care of your heart by changing to become a first-timer.

Ways to Change

Make a plan of attack to cross that line and break through the roadblocks. Start building a support network of people who will help you: a training buddy, a personal trainer, a coach, a mentor, anybody who can help chart your progress. Enroll in a group exercise program, or buy some home exercise equipment with a video to help you learn how to use it properly. Read more on fitness training, and subscribe to a sports participation magazine. Ask a friend to start a fitness-training program, and get going together. If you experience a relapse, use it as a learning experience. Recommit to a new plan, regroup, and go at it. We all have setbacks, so prepare for one or more. If necessary, allow yourself more flexibility in the plan to accommodate the unexpected. If the plan isn't working, change the plan, not the work. Go to a sports event for amateurs as a spectator and see what kinds of people are achieving all kinds of small wonders in their lives. The people at the back of the pack are always the most interesting and the most inspirational. Ask yourself, "Could I do that?" The answer is always "yes."

Activities for Moving Up

You have found a physical activity that you enjoy. Think of it as a new challenge, something to learn more about. Join a basketball, softball, or volleyball recreation team. Buy the uniform. Pay the dues. Attend the workouts. You are not going to be the best player on the team when you begin, but you are now a player and you have a team. Go to the practices. Start to work out to get in shape for the sport. Ask the coach or manager of the team for exercises you can do at home that can help you be a better player. Invite one of the other players on the team to practice with you and be your mentor. By constantly improving, just small improvements, playing gets easier. The fitter you are, the better your playing skills will be and the more you will enjoy it. Take it slow, and don't have high expectations at first; just keep going to the practices and getting better at the game.

Step 4: The First-Timer

You are training regularly. This is a time when continued motivational activities are essential to staying in the game. Setting and working toward goals is very important at this point. Changing from a first-timer to a regular player is a matter of staying on the program and staying in the game.

Ways to Change

Use your health club membership or get access to exercise equipment to keep you motivated and getting fitter. Enroll in several group workout classes; most of us train better when we are with others at the same level. Write a contract with yourself to exercise a minimum of 30 minutes a day most days. Give yourself some rewards for accomplishing your goals. Personal commitment to the program makes it work. This is the time for self-motivation, like feeling stronger emotionally, physically, and metabolically. Search for the training program that you enjoy the most. Keep a training log. Get a role model. Provide yourself with incentives and rewards. Get support from your friends.

Activities for Moving Up

You now have a workout plan. As an example, your plan might include physical activity 5 times a week for 30 to 45 minutes. Use your heart rate monitor for every workout, and stay in the low training zones, zones 1 to 3. Warm up in zone 1 and use zones 2 and 3 for your main set. Vary your workouts. One day walk; the next day, swim or bike. This is called cross-training. Include strength training at home or at a club at least two times a week. Stretch on a daily basis so you maintain your range of motion. Look for more energy-shifting activities, such as taking the stairs instead of the elevator at the office or in a shopping center.

Step 5: The Athlete

You are dedicated to lifelong fitness training. This is the best place to be, and you made it. Continue to get fitter by playing and learning more about the Fit *and* Fat Training Program using heart zones training.

Ways to Change

Do some sports events regularly, like walking events, triathlons, hiking challenges, cycle touring, and other activities that challenge you. Spend your holidays with like-minded people and get fired up about your sport. Try a new angle of your sport or branch out. Learn more about your heart rate by keeping a careful log of your training activities and your performances. Find an aspect of your sport that your spouse, partner, or kids can enjoy, too, or try something new together.

Activities for Moving Up

Get several different training partners. Set a specific workout schedule with them. Increase your workout time by 10 percent a week for the next month. It's time for you to become a mentor to someone who is a spectator or a speculator. You can teach that person what you know about training. You get better at training by showing someone else how and why to do it. You can write your own workouts. Use the examples in this book of training in different zones on different days to get different benefits.

From Spectator to Athlete

With your current stage of fitness training in mind, remember that you need to move forward step by step. Go from spectator to speculator, not spectator to athlete, progressing slowly and surely from one stage of change to the next.

At first Kelly Cantrell saw herself as a sideliner. A year later, she had moved through first-timer to athlete. Her individual program, her support team, her training partners, and her realistic goals kept her motivated every step of the way.

Motivation fuels the fitness engine. The higher your level of self-motivation is, the easier you will find it to keep going when the going gets tough. Highly motivated people build immunity from the "drop-out bug." How do you immunize yourself? Unfortunately, it's not easy, but with planning you can do it.

Unlike readiness to change, self-motivation does not follow a simple progression from low to high. It's much more individual than that, and more something that you are born with, part of your personality. For example, few of us could muster the extreme levels of self-motivation needed to ski across Antarctica while enduring tremendous personal hardship. Some people perform best solo; others perform best in harmony with a team. In addition, motivation depends on your level of interest. Perhaps you can catch the vision of sailing but not of hiking. The bottom line? Your specific personality dictates how you motivate yourself. That's another reason why you need to design a unique program. Don't make it harder for yourself by creating a program that calls for high levels of self-motivation you can't maintain. Never create barriers to fitness. You'll hit enough walls as it is.

Activity 8.2: Put Your Motivation into Your Plan

Read each of the following statements and ask yourself to what extent each statement applied to me.

1. I can persevere at stressful tasks, even when they are physically tiring or painful.

2. I have a lot of willpower. If I've said I'll do something you can be sure I'll get it done.

3. It takes a lot to get me going and I get discouraged easily.

4. I'm just not the goal-setting type; I prefer to be spontaneous.

5. I can persist despite failure and I have a strong desire to achieve.

How did you fare on these five questions? Do you think you are the type of person with a high level of self-motivation or does your lack of motivation sometimes let you down? It doesn't matter whether you are self-motivated or not, you can build your fitness program around whatever level your own motivational characteristics. Based on whether you think your levels of self-motivation are very low, somewhat

Activity 8.2. *continued*

low, moderate, high, or very high, the following are some ways you can structure your fitness plan to accommodate your motivational profile. Read through the tips for your category of motivation and note any ideas that could work for you in your personal fitness log.

Very low to extremely low. Your fitness plan must include the following elements to ensure success:

- It's very important for your program to be initiated by you. You design it and choose what you want to do and when.

- You will need lots of help and encouragement to stick with the program. Most workout sessions should include a trainer or supervisor to ensure that you actually carry out the workout. Consider joining a program, as long as it fits in with what you want to do, so that you can receive high levels of personal attention and support.

- Enlist your family and friends, and tell them you need their encouragement to maintain fitness as a priority in your life. Recognize each small achievement and tell others about it.

- Set up a reward system. Focus on implementing very small but permanent changes in your life.

- Find somebody who made the same journey, and ask that person to give you positive reinforcement and encouragement.

Somewhat low. Your fitness plan must include doing a lot of different things that help you overcome low levels of motivation:

- Join a group of people with similar fitness goals, or find training partners.

- A mentor, personal trainer, or coach can help.

- Arrange your fitness sessions in advance, making it harder to back out at the last minute.

- Consider working with animals as a way to get motivated (dogs and horses are ideal).

- Consider sports that require teamwork or that incorporate other skills, such as orienteering, which combines navigational skills and physical fitness.

- Try sports that have a structured progression system (golf or fencing). If it could be a barrier to participation take care not to select activities that require either the purchase of expensive equipment or a high level of competence before you get fitness benefits. On the other hand, investing in a new fitness toy could be just the stimulus you need. Be very careful not to make your program too demanding or challenging at first.

Moderate. Consider tricks to help you stay self-motivated.

- Purchase a membership or season ticket to a sports facility instead of paying individually for each visit. This will encourage you to use the facility more.
- Find a training buddy who's a stickler for regular appointments.
- Buy some new exercise clothes or equipment. Join a new club, or try something new you think you will enjoy.
- Consider sports that take you to a new environment and that could fire up your imagination, such as diving or caving.
- Rely on a mentor or coach to keep you on the right track and give you new ideas.

High. You could benefit from setting yourself some challenging goals.

- Find people in your sport who have been highly successful, and get to know them. Get some advice or training in technical aspects of your activity.
- Structure your training and regularly check your progress.
- Help others who are not as experienced as you. You'll both benefit.

Very high to extremely high. Set challenging goals. You are confident in training and competing and are ready to test yourself to the limit.

- Find out what hasn't been done before in your sport, and make that your own unique challenge.
- Use your levels of motivation to effect change in other people's lives by offering your help to the less experienced or motivated. Allow others to celebrate your achievements.

When Kelly completed the preceding questionnaire, she found herself in the moderate range, so she needed to develop ways to boost and retain higher motivation levels. Here's what she did:

- Joined Team Danskin Training, a group just for women wanting to complete a Danskin triathlon.
- Got a mentor. She found Suzanne, an experienced triathlete who helped Kelly train and gave her encouragement.
- Signed up for a coached swim program. Having paid the money for the six-week course up front, Kelly found herself more motivated to turn up for the weekly session and do her "home-work," swimming by herself twice a week.
- Told her two sisters what she wanted to accomplish and discussed her progress with them once a week.

Obstacles and Roadblocks

You will want to forecast other factors that may influence your ability to succeed in your quest for fitness. Any number of obstacles or roadblocks can pop up. Injury, illness, loss of a job, the start of a new job, and disruptions in our personal lives, from the birth of a baby to the death of a loved one—all can present temporary obstacles on the road to fitness. But if you can anticipate them you will find them easier to deal with them, especially if you enjoy the support of others.

Activity 8.3: Forecasting the Odds

What obstacles and roadblocks might you encounter on the road to fitness? Are the odds of achieving success stacked for you or against you? The following table lists some common obstacles such as your social support, your level of self-belief, and the amount of discomfort you feel when you exercise. Anticipating obstacles is the first step toward overcoming them. If you know the odds, you can beat them.

Each of the responses to the following failure-factor questions is weighted on a scale from 1 (low) to 6 (high). Check the box next to the number of your response for each of the following:

A. *Do your friends fitness-train?*

- ❏ 1 All my friends train regularly and encourage me to train with them.
- ❏ 2 Most of my friends train or take part in recreational fitness activities.
- ❏ 3 Many of the people I know train regularly in one way or another.

❑ 4 I know some people who participate in regular fitness activities.

❑ 5 Few people I know do sports or physical training other than that required for their daily lives.

❑ 6 Nobody I know currently takes part in any active fitness training or sports.

B. Do you believe you can do it?

❑ 1 Yes, I'm confident I can achieve anything I set my mind to.

❑ 2 Probably. I usually get there in the end, even if I take a little longer than I thought I would.

❑ 3 I think I can do it if I get the right kind of preparation and learn a few new skills.

❑ 4 Maybe I can do it. I can see it's going to be hard, but maybe it will be all right if I manage to learn the new skills and get ready in time.

❑ 5 I'm worried that I've bitten off more than I can chew.

❑ 6 I'm afraid it's a huge task; I don't know where to start. I've failed before, and I'm afraid of failing again.

C. Are your friends, family, and colleagues supporting you?

❑ 1 Yes, my partner, family, and friends encourage me to train by asking me to join them.

❑ 2 They do encourage me and are supportive, but sometimes other priorities get in the way.

❑ 3 I think my family and friends would be supportive if I told them what I wanted to do and why.

❑ 4 Because few of my friends and family train, it's difficult for them to understand what it's all about, and I feel a bit isolated.

❑ 5 Not only do people not understand, but they are making no effort to understand, and that discourages me.

❑ 6 People actively discourage me, saying I'm too fat/too old/too unfit to be training.

D. Do you experience physical discomfort when you fitness-train?

❏ 1 No, I love training and I get a real high from it. It's the best part of my day, and I can't wait to get out there.

❏ 2 I love training and feel great.

❏ 3 I enjoy it, but only afterward. It's not painful or uncomfortable, but I feel better afterward.

❏ 4 I do feel some pain during fitness training.

❏ 5 I find most exercise mildly uncomfortable. I get too hot and too sticky, find it hard to breathe, and can't wait for it to end. Afterward, my limbs ache, so it's hard to feel good about exercising.

❏ 6 Physical exercise causes me so much discomfort that it forces me to stop the activity. My skin chaps, my whole body wobbles and shakes, my legs and knees ache, and I really dread it. How can something that feels so awful really be good for me?

E. Do you use tobacco?

❏ 1 I am a nonsmoker.

❏ 2 I occasionally smoke a cigar or pipe.

❏ 3 I smoke 10 or fewer cigarettes daily.

❏ 4 I smoke 20 cigarettes a day.

❏ 5 I smoke 30 cigarettes a day.

❏ 6 I smoke 40 or more cigarettes a day.

F. How would you describe your body image?

❏ 1 I don't even think about my body image: I feel confident exercising in any setting, even before an audience.

❏ 2 I'm proud of my body for what it does and how it looks. I'm happy to display it in a fitness-training setting.

❏ 3 I feel fairly happy about my body and don't mind exercising with other people who accept me as I am.

❏ 4 I know my body image affects my choices about where and when to train. For example, I avoid swimming when there are kids in the pool, and I can't imagine taking part in sports in which people wear revealing outfits.

❑ 5 I find it hard to relax and enjoy fitness training with people who are fitter or slimmer than me.

❑ 6 I'm really embarrassed about my body. It's hard for me to enjoy training with other people because I'm so self-conscious. I find it intimidating to use communal changing or showering facilities.

If you scored 3 or greater in any of the failure-factor questions, you should think about making changes that will decrease the odds of this factor affecting your chances of success. For each of the odds in which you scored 3 or greater, try these suggestions for modifying your program to increase your odds of success:

- **I don't know anybody who trains.** Actively seek out people who have been in the same situation as you and successfully made changes in their lives. If you can't find any near where you live, try the Internet.

- **I don't believe I can do it.** Break the task into manageable chunks so that the task immediately in front of you is always something you know you can achieve. Try to find other people who you identify with who have achieved what you want to achieve: If they can do it, then maybe you can, too.

- **Friends and family do not support me.** Explain to your support network what you are doing, how important it is to you, and what you need each person to do. For example, you may need somebody to baby-sit for two hours a week to allow you to fitness-train. You may need your colleague to stop making fun of your biking outfit you commute to work in. You may need your training buddy to call you in the morning to make sure you awaken on time.

- **I smoke a lot.** Try to stop smoking. Realize how important it is not just because of the health risks of smoking itself, but also because it prevents you from gaining the benefits of fitness.

- **I find exercise uncomfortable.** Consult a physician about any specific medical problems, and make it clear that you want assistance to enable you to continue exercising. Think of ways to get around the discomfort. Can you try a different sport that gives you less discomfort, such as swimming or indoor cycling? Try sports gels or creams designed to reduce chafing. Research the

Activity 8.3. *continued*

best types of fabrics for your skin and manufacturers that offer specialized workout clothing in your size. Take steps to reduce discomfort after exercising, such as doing a thorough cooldown, taking a sauna or warm/cold bath, having a massage, and using ice on sore spots. If you're female and feel that everything is wobbling around when you exercise, consider the use of sports clothing with built-in foundation support, such as that produced for maternity wear, to reduce discomfort. For feet, knee, or hip aches and pains, consider gait analysis and advice on footwear. Consider consulting a physical therapist for persistent aches and pains. If discomfort persists, consider restricting the aerobic training aspect of your program and concentrating on strength, flexibility, and metabolic and emotional fitness until you feel more comfortable.

- **I have a negative body image.** Fitness-train at home using a workout video until you gain more confidence. Find a class in which the instructor and other participants are of a similar body type/size. Set aside time and a budget to acquire sports clothing that makes you feel more comfortable. Talk to somebody about your worries, especially other people your size who appear more confident. If you are considering taking part in a new activity, observe it beforehand to make sure you will feel comfortable exercising in that setting. Take a friend along the first time.

Here's how Kelly decided to reduce the odds stacked against her:

- **Do your friends fitness-train?** "I scored a 4 on this one because I don't know many people who have trained for a triathlon. Most of my friends thought I was crazy. When I joined the Danskin training group, I immediately found lots of people who had trained, and this encouraged me enormously."

- **Do you believe you can do it?** "I scored a 3 because I really did think I could do it. I looked at my swimming and thought I needed to be able to swim only twice as far as I can right now, so each week I increased the distance just a little bit. Biking? Well, I knew I could ride a bike. Didn't know how fast, but that wasn't really an issue, since all I wanted to do was finish the race. Think about speed later. Running was my biggest worry. I really didn't know whether I could run 2.5 miles, but I knew I could gradually improve if I took it step by step. My first goal was to run for 5 minutes without stopping."

- **Are your friends and family and colleagues supporting you?** "I explained to my children and husband that this was something I really wanted to do. My kids thought it was a great idea and told all their friends about it, who told their moms, who then kept asking me how it was going. My husband was supportive, as he'd run several marathons himself and knew what it was all about. It was harder, though, for him to get home on time for me to get to my swim lessons, but he usually managed it just in time."

- **Do you experience physical discomfort when you fitness-train?** "I scored a 4 because one of the reasons I don't like running is the feeling of everything wobbling around. The girls at the training group introduced me to sport bras that helped. I also did some strength training that seemed to anchor everything down. I also got some new sports clothing that made me feel sportier."

- **Do you use tobacco?** "I don't smoke."

- **How would you describe your body image?** "I also scored a 4 here, but I improved rapidly. I found a training group with lots of other women my size, and suddenly it seemed not to matter half as much. They showed me what I could wear in the triathlon to feel comfortable with my body, and it became less and less of an issue."

What Are Your Priorities?

Do you ever feel like you're going as fast as you can but making no headway? You feel time-starved and hurried, with each day blending into the next in a gray blur? Well, that happens to us all these days, but when it does, I always try to tell myself to pause, take a deep breath, and look around. Imagine you're a child crossing a busy street. Wouldn't you stop and look both ways before stepping off the curb? The same holds true for fitness training and discovering the athlete inside.

It's human nature to want instant results, but fitness results come only gradually and progressively. You can't jog two miles, go to bed, and wake up fit the next morning. Training for metabolic, physical, and emotional fitness takes time. So take a little time now, pausing before you step into the street to conduct a few simple fitness assessments, which will help guide you to a program that will help you set the right priorities for you.

Activity 8.4: Identifying Your Priorities

In order to set your priorities, rate each of the following three on a scale of 1 to 10:

Set Priorities

Fitness	Importance to You	Your Element Score
Metabolic fitness	I'm metabolically fit, so I'm not really concerned about metabolic fitness.	My physician has told me that I must improve my metabolic fitness or my health will suffer.

1   2   3   4   5   6   7   8   9   10

Emotional fitness	I'm emotionally fit, so I don't need to make any special adjustments to my current mind/body regime.	I've recognized major emotional areas of my life that would benefit from emotional fitness training. If I don't do something about them, they soon will adversely affect my health.

1   2   3   4   5   6   7   8   9   10

Physical fitness	I'm physically fit, so I don't need further enhancements as long as I stick to my program.	I need to make a major commitment to physical fitness because my life depends on it.

1   2   3   4   5   6   7   8   9   10

Divide each score by your total score (the three added together), and multiply each by 100 to find the percentage of your time you should spend on that particular element. For example, Kelly's scores were 4 for metabolic fitness, 3 for emotional fitness, and 7 for physical fitness. Because her three scores added up to 14, Kelly's percentages worked out as follows:

Metabolic fitness: $4 \div 14 = .29 \times 100 = 29$ percent

Emotional fitness: $3 \div 14 = .21 \times 100 = 21$ percent

Physical fitness: $7 \div 14 = .50 \times 100 = 50$ percent

Goals for the Game of Life

Every fitness program requires goals. Yes, you have set general goals concerning your need for metabolic, emotional, and physical fitness, but you must also establish more specific and exact goals that can help you mark your progress and keep you motivated. Again, scientific research by physical fitness professionals has found a strong correlation between fitness-training success and goals:[3]

- Individuals with goals achieve more.
- Goals work best when they are measurable over a set period of time.
- Results improve when you rank multiple goals in terms of relative importance.
- Short-term and intermediate goals more surely lead to attaining the ultimate goal.
- A plan of action facilitates goal attainment.
- Flexible goals work better than rigid ones.
- Publicly acknowledged goals work better than secret goals.

Goals provide both motivation and a yardstick to measure progress. Just wishing for success won't make it happen. No, you need to wish for something very specific and concrete: "I want to train to the point that I can comfortably complete a 5k road race." You can't just say, "I want a rich, happy, and productive life." Instead, you must get specific and say, "I want to lower my blood pressure, cholesterol numbers, and blood sugar levels, and I want to deal with stress more effectively." The former only stimulates vague motivation and gives you nothing to measure, while the latter strongly motivates you to make measurable progress.

It's even better to add a time element. "I want to run that 5k race three months from now." Now you can make your progress week by week until you cross that finish line on October 15. Specific goals, measurable goals, and goals broken into time-specific segments all add up to a plan. You can't win the game of life without a plan of attack. And go public! Tell everybody who supports you about your goal, and you'll instantly enlist 50 people rooting for you to succeed.

Activity 8.5: Setting Your Goals

A goal originates from a dream. It's about the things you always really wanted to do, the way you always wanted to live your life but were too busy or weak or scared to make a primary priority. Promise yourself now that you will recapture your dreams and turn them into realities in your life. Set your goals today.

Spend some quiet time by yourself, perhaps taking a long walk, meditating in a quiet room, soaking in a fragrant bath, or gazing out to sea. Empty your mind of all your prior conditioning and experiences. Forget for a moment who you are.

Activity 8.5. *continued*

Who do you want to become? How did you imagine your adult life when you were a child? Do you still want what you imagined, or do you want something else? Dig deep inside yourself, freeing yourself from the context of your current lifestyle and situation. Do you long for strength and stamina, a strong body to walk up mountains and trek across plains, to cycle across continents, to swim across oceans, to ride breaking waves, or even to fly in the sky? Do you dream of sprinting the hurdles, running in a stadium with fans cheering your athletic prowess, or crossing the finish line of a marathon? Have you done those things? Do you wish you still could do them? Do you feel constrained by the limitations of your body? Have you managed to access the extraordinary power of the athlete within? What would your life feel like if you could? Would you feel more confident, powerful, and satisfied, a master of the gravity, friction, and the wild environments of our planet?

Release the vision of who you would like to become, how it would feel as your body carried you up that mountain, across that tightrope, through the choppy waters of that lake. Now connect with your everyday life. What element of your dream could you add to your current life to capture even a little bit of this dream? Since you know you can't have it all at once, pick just one aspect, like learning to skate across ice in a perfect glide, hitting a tennis ball to exactly where you want it on the court, or cutting past your opponents to cleanly dunk a basket. Write that down.

Next, break down your goal into manageable chunks. After all, your goal comes from a dream, and dreams live in far-off places that it takes weeks, months, even years to reach. Here's how you do it:

- Set up stakes or milestones. Imagine that a goal is like a stake in the ground. Place two or more stakes between today and the achievement of your goal. A 4-week goal might require 2 to 4 stages, while a 3-month goal might require 12 or more. Remember, take it slow and easy.

- Specify your stakes. Give each a date and a specific accomplishment. If your stake is the fifth one toward the tenth that marks running 3 miles, you might label it: "Run 1.5 miles on or about June 17."

- Formulate a strategy. Determine exactly how you are going to get to each stake and what will get you to the final stake.

- Be sensible. Set a realistic and practical goal, something within your reach. Notice how Lorraine began with something she really could do in a reasonable amount of time. Achieving the possible goal strengthens and motivates you toward what otherwise seems an impossible goal.

- Be strong. Back yourself up with your strongest personal commitment. Commitment gives you strength, a power and life force that will propel you steadily forward.

Here's how Kelly structured her goal in a winning way. Use the form in Appendix F to write down and structure your own goal.

The Five S's of Goal Setting

S1—Stakes	Ultimate goal: To finish my first triathlon.
	Stake 1: Double the longest distance I can swim to half a mile.
	Stake 2: Complete two practice swims in open water.
	Stake 3: Learn to run.
	Stake 4: Ride my bike continuously for 12 miles.
	Stake 5: Do a sprint triathlon (0.5 mile swimming, 12 miles biking, 3.1 miles running).
S2—Specificity	Stake 1: By July 21, 2002.
	Stake 2: On vacation July 2 to 5, 2002.
	Stake 3: Be able to run/walk 3 miles by July 21, 2002.
	Stake 4: Be able to ride 12 miles by July 21, 2002.
	Stake 5: My first triathlon will be August 4, 2002, at Cherry Creek, Denver Colorado.
S3—Strategy	Stake 1: Sign up for a Masters Swim Course.
	Stake 2: Ask my husband to reserve some time to help me with the swim.
	Stake 3: Use my heart rate monitor to walk or run in Zone 3.
	Stake 4: Ride on the weekends for one to two hours. Have my husband service my bike.
	Stake 5: Sign up now and tell all my friends and family.
S4—Sensibility	Stake 1: Talk to the trainer about how much she thinks I can improve.

Activity 8.5. *continued*

                Stake 2: Do the practice swims only if somebody is watching me.

                Stake 3: Use my heart rate monitor to keep the intensity manageable and not get injured by overdoing it: I'm going to stick in Zone 3 for now.

                Stake 4: I think this is manageable; I just need to extend a little bit.

                Stake 5: It's a big and scary objective, but I know women who've done it, so I'm going to give it a shot.

S5—Strength   I really want to achieve this goal and can see how each step is crucial to achieving the final goal. For years, I have supported my husband and kids doing all sorts of amazing things. Now it's my turn. I have this vision of how fantastic I will feel if I can finish the race: That's what I want, and that's why I am doing it. I also want the health benefits of becoming fitter, and having a goal like this might finally help me to get fit.

Kelly used this approach to help her to get not only to the starting line of her final stake, the triathlon, but also to all the ones in between. Kelly crossed that finish line listening to the screams of the thousands of spectators who came to cheer the finishers and celebrate their accomplishment with them. Her dream came true: She became a triathlete. Following your own Fit *and* Fat Personal Activity Program can make yours come true, too.

Putting It All Together

Finally, you can put together all that you've learned about fitness in general and about your specific makeup and needs to commit your unique personal plan to paper. It will get the results you seek because ...

- You yourself create and control it.
- It reflects your own personal commitment to change, self-motivation, and understanding of the odds stacked against you.
- It follows your fitness priorities.
- It aims at reasonable and achievable goals that you set.

Activity 8.6: Completing Your Personal Fitness Plan Profile

To capture all the crucial information you need for your plan, transcribe the results of the activities you've completed so far in this chapter into your personal fitness plan profile. Use the form in Appendix F. Here is what Kelly's looked like.

Personal Fitness Plan Profile

Activity	Kelly's Results	Elements to Include in Your Fitness Program
The five steps of fitness change (Activity 8.1)	Sideliner	I want to get fit and realize the benefits I'll gain if I can manage it. I need to make up a program, rally my support team, find some training partners, and set some goals.
Self-motivation inventory (Activity 8.2)	Moderately self-motivated	• Join Team Danskin, a training group just for women training to complete a Danskin triathlon. • Get a mentor. • Sign up for a coached swim program. • Tell my sisters what I am doing and ask them to call me weekly.
Forecasting the odds (Activity 8.3)	Friends 4 Self-belief 3 Support 3	Join the Team Danskin training group. Set up a number of small goals for running. Talk to my husband and children. Ask my husband to be home early on Tuesdays and Thursdays so I can go swimming.
	Smoking 1 Discomfort 4	I don't smoke. Investigate sports bras and new sports clothing.
	Body image 4	I need to meet other women of my body size/type who've trained and completed a triathlon.
Identifying priorities (Activity 8.4)	Metabolic training: 30 percent of my time Emotional training: 20 percent of my time Physical training: 50 percent of my time	

The information you completed this table with forms the basis for the next activity. Now you have all the information assembled to enable you to draw up your own individual weekly training schedule. Work through the steps of the following activity to build your personal activity program.

Activity 8.7: Building Your Own Fit *and* Fat Personal Activity Program

Now it's time to assemble all the pieces into a concrete program. At the end of this activity, you will have written a program with scheduled times for your different workouts and types of training. It requires only five easy steps. Use the protocol provided in Appendix F.

1. **Set the time.** How much time can you devote to working toward your goal per week?

    i) The number of days a week I can train: _____

    ii) The amount of time I can devote to training each day: _____

    My total weekly training time i) × ii) = _____

    Kelly decided that she could train five days a week for one hour each day, for a total of five hours per week.

2. **Manage your time.** Look at your results from Activity 8.4. Divide your total amount of time among metabolic, emotional, and fitness training, according to your priorities.

    Kelly's looked like this:

Type of Fitness Training	Percent of Your Time to Allocate to This Type of Training	Actual Time Allocated to This Type of Training
Metabolic	30 percent	1.5 hours
Emotional	20 percent	1 hour
Physical	50 percent	2.5 hours

3. **Select your activities.** Now you can consider the kinds of activities that will enable you to achieve your training objectives. If you've set a goal to run a certain distance, then your metabolic activities might include slow running; your physical activity might include aerobic or interval running, and strength training and stretching after running and on rest days. For emotional fitness training, you might read a book about a famous runner who inspires you. If your goal is to perform a flamenco dance, your metabolic training might be learning new steps, your physical training might be some swimming to improve your overall muscle tone, and your emotional fitness training might be spending time socializing with your dancing partners.

Look at Kelly's choices:

Type of Fitness Training	Activities
Metabolic	Swim coaching
Physical	Running
	Swim training
	Strength-training video
Emotional	Meeting with Team Danskin.
	Biking outing with my kids.

4. **Choose the best time.** When can you best carry out each of the different types of training you've chosen? For example, you might be able to fit in swimming in the morning, but you can do dance practice only in the evenings on Tuesdays and Thursdays. Perhaps your running partner prefers to run between 7 P.M. and 8 P.M. This table will pinpoint when you can do the activities you've selected.

Here's how Kelly did it:

Type of Fitness Training	Selected Activities	Schedule
Metabolic	Swim coaching	Tuesdays 6:30 to 7:30 P.M.
Physical	Running	Mornings 6:30 to 7 A.M.
	Swim training	Friday and Sunday evenings 8 to 9 P.M.
	Strength training—video	Mornings 6:30 to 7 A.M.
Emotional	Meeting with Team Danskin	Fridays 7 to 8 P.M.
	Biking outing with my kids	Saturday or Sunday

5. **Assemble your program.** To complete your program, use a weekly planner and fill in what you are going to do and when. Include any information about where you are going to do the workout, with whom, and at what heart rate. Include a final column so that you can mark whether you did the workout and how it went.

―Activity 8.7. *continued*―

Here's what Kelly's weekly planner looked like:

Day	Time	Workout	Additional Details: Type of Workout, Where, with Whom, Any Special Notes	Log: How Was the Workout?
Monday	6:30 to 7 A.M.	Running	Meet with Jane from Team Danskin, Zones 1 and 2 running.	
Tuesday	6:30 to 7:30 P.M.	Swim coaching		
Wednesday	6:30 to 7:30 P.M.	Running	Zone 3 running.	
Thursday	6:30 to 7 A.M.	Strength training	Use my home video.	
Friday	8 to 8:45 P.M.	Swim practice	Practice what I learned on Tuesday.	
Saturday	Rest day			
Sunday	10 to 11 A.M.	Biking with the family		
	8 to 8:45 P.M.	Swim	Try a longer swim practice using my new techniques. Increase the distance a little every week.	

Week 7 Summary

This week, you put all the pieces of your program together to build your own personalized Fit *and* Fat Training Program. You've uniquely tailored it to your dreams and needs. You've assessed your levels of motivation and built the program around your own specific goals. You learned how Kelly built up her program and used it to achieve her goal of finishing her first triathlon. You, too, can achieve success if you faithfully follow your own program. In the next chapter, I supply you with more tricks to help you stick to it, get back on board if you fall off, and keep motivated. Can you feel that athlete inside cheering you on?

CHAPTER 9

Week 8: Motivation Magic

Staying the Course for Life

Just where do some people get their motivation? We all know them: they are the people we just can't believe what they've been up to and achieved. Do you think they were born with it or did they somehow learn it? Well, the good news is that to a large extent you *can* learn how to keep yourself well motivated. Keeping a positive mental attitude will help you succeed not just on your Fit *and* Fat Personal Activity Program but in all aspects of your life. This week, as you try out the first week of the program you built last week, read about how to acquire some key motivational skills, like how to reframe your mental approach to obstacles.

Where Do Some People Get It?: Jeanette's Story

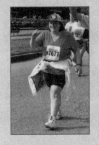 *One of my favorite stories about superhuman motivation involves Jeanette DePatie, a marketing consultant who runs her own firm in Missouri. Jeanette had always thought of herself as "just a fat person." But without becoming any less of a fat person, she transformed herself into a triathlete, marathoner, certified aerobics instructor, and owner of a fitness business. She even produced a fitness video titled* The Fat Chick Works Out *that has landed her a number of television appearances. In her own words:*

I remember the day quite clearly. I was in the kitchen with my husband, and I was crying inconsolably. I was crying because I was fat, and I believed being fat was cause to be miserable. My husband assured me that I looked great. He told me he loved me just the way I was. The sad thing was, I couldn't believe him. He told me he would help me any way he could. He would diet with me; he would exercise with me, anything. And he did. I lost a little bit of weight, but I was still miserable.

Fast forward to another day much later when I was in Springfield, Missouri, with my friend Mary Ann about to cross the finish line of my first marathon. It was quiet. There was no finish line to speak of (they had taken it down hours earlier). But I limped across the sidewalk where the finish line had been, raised my exhausted arms in victory, and sobbed like a baby. But this time, they were tears of joy. Mary Ann and I cried together as we celebrated my first-ever marathon finish.

Another day, later still. The heat was unbelievable in our makeshift video studio. It was at least 96 degrees in there. My friends Nora, Mary Ellen, and Mary Ann and I had been doing aerobics for over four hours, shooting footage for my new exercise video (*The Fat Chick Works Out*).

So how did it happen? How did I motivate myself to evolve from that pathetic, sobbing creature at the kitchen table to a triathlete, marathoner, certified aerobics instructor, and fitness celebrity who proudly calls herself "The Fat Chick"?

Actually, a lot of things happened during that time of conversion. But it started with one little idea that changed everything. It was a simple idea and, in retrospect, a totally obvious one. But when I first entertained it, I was stunned. I was flabbergasted. It hit me like a bolt out of the blue. It was very simply, "What if I stop obsessing about how to lose weight and start living my life as if I already had?"

It was a revolutionary concept. I stopped weighing and measuring every morsel of food that went into my mouth. No more exchanges. No more points. No more food journal. No more weighing myself. No more measuring my worth in terms of a number on a scale.

I began to live my life as if I were already thin. There were so many things I wanted to do after I lost weight. I wanted new clothes. I wanted a new hairdo. I wanted to teach aerobics classes. I wanted to be on TV. I suddenly decided that I would stop wasting my life while minding my waist. And I would start living the life of my dreams right now.

Frankly, I didn't come to that decision all by myself. One day, I was in the library looking for yet another "solve all your problems, lose weight in a week" diet book. I accidentally picked up Laura Fraser's book *Losing It in America*. In this scathing expose on the diet industry, I finally heard an obviously smart and successful woman saying what my heart knew all along: that I was okay now. I should stop wasting my time and money on things that don't matter and start enjoying my life. I will always be grateful to Ms. Fraser, both for the message in her book and for introducing me to the National Association to Advance Fat Acceptance (NAAFA).

Finding the people at NAAFA unquestionably changed my life. Ten days after I learned of the existence of this organization, NAAFA was holding its national convention. I went to talk to my husband. We were pretty broke at the time, and any extra trips would mean that we couldn't go on a vacation together that year. I asked my husband what he thought I should do. He took one look at the excitement shining in my eyes and said "Go." (He still submits that this is the best investment we ever made.) Before I knew it, I was on a plane to Los Angeles.

The NAAFA national convention simply blew my mind. Here were hundreds of fat people wearing swimsuits, dancing, sharing, exercising, learning, partying down, and just living. I took one look at what these people had and decided, "I want that." I was finally free.

When I got back, I went to the local YWCA and told them that I wanted to become an aerobics instructor. Frankly, some people looked at me funny. Several said that it wasn't a good idea. I almost gave up. Then I met Ahmena, a loving, beautiful, joyful black woman who taught aerobics at the Y. She also happened to be fat. I am so grateful to her. She taught me the mechanics of teaching a successful aerobics class. What's more, she never doubted for one second that I could do it. Before long, I was teaching a class of my own.

I learned an awful lot from teaching aerobics. One thing I learned was that when you separate fitness training from the expectation of weight loss, it is really fun! I discovered that I loved it! And for the first time in my life, I really appreciated what exercise could do for me. I slept well. I felt great. Stress just melted away. I also saw what exercise did for my students. Some lost weight. Some didn't. Some got off diabetes medication or blood pressure medication. Some found they could run up to our second-floor studio without huffing and puffing. Some found a new, bolder, and braver sense of self. Some simply found a way to spend an hour away from family obligations to take care of themselves. There was something for everybody. Ultimately, I became a certified aerobics instructor and personal trainer.

But I didn't stop there. One New Year's Eve, my husband I went to dinner with Jeff and Mary Ann. It was an eight-course dinner with very good wine. We drank a *lot* of wine. Mary Ann mentioned that she always wanted to do a marathon. "Me, too!" I cried. (Did I mention there was a lot of wine?) By the time the fruit and cheese and midnight champagne arrived, Mary Ann and I had made a pact to do a marathon together. She was with me every step of the way for 26.2 miles. The training was hard.

Finishing was grueling. But it was one of the most spectacular moments of my life. I am so grateful to Mary Ann for helping me get there.

During my hundreds of hours of training that year, I had a lot of time to think. I reflected on all the people who had helped me cross that finish line. I thought of Mary Ann, Ahmena, Laura Fraser, all the folks at NAAFA, my family, and my wonderful husband. I thought of what their loving support meant to me. And I thought of a way to lend that support to other beginning exercisers. I currently serve as a media coordinator and NAAFA spokeswoman. In this role, I have done many interviews on radio, on television, and in print, encouraging people to stop waiting to enjoy and live their lives. I am also putting my life experiences to work on a brand new exercise DVD called *The Fat Chick Works Out*. I hope through this project to give support to people everywhere who want to work out but have been discouraged by their imperfections. It's a big job, but that's okay. I'm a big girl.

You can learn about NAAFA at www.naafa.org, and you can preview and purchase Jeanette's workout DVD at www.thefatchick.com.

Conquering Resistance to Change

Jeanette realized a moment of motivation magic when she made the simple decision to change an attitude that had been holding her back. It wasn't easy. Permanent changes in your life, whether they relate to your weight, your lifestyle, your daily routine, or even your emotional life, are always hard to make. It's not so much a reflection on our lack of willpower as it is the difficulty of making changes over the long term.

Humans are biologically programmed to resist change, a phenomenon scientists call homeostasis, a feedback system that operates to maintain consistency in human systems. We see homeostatic systems at work in all aspects of our lives, from our genes, our metabolism, and our physical selves, to our emotional lives, our work communities, our society, and even world order. Any action that tries to change any part of any one of these systems will meet with homeostatic resistance. Biology doesn't like change and wants us to stay just like we are. Biology is all about survival. If we are surviving, our biology says, "Why fix something that ain't broken?" That's the one flaw with homeostasis: It can't tell a good change from a bad change; it resists all change equally. Homeostasis will resist all of your attempts to make good changes in your life. So prepare yourself for resistance. It's natural.

The principle holds that our bodies and brains have a built-in tendency to keep things the same, sometimes within quite narrow boundaries. Take temperature, for example. The regulation of our body's temperature involves the skin, the nervous system, the brain, and behavior. The skin's temperature sensors send messages to the brain, which processes the information and decides what to do about it. The brain then sends out nerve impulses that stimulate corrective responses. If we get too hot, these responses may include increased sweating and dilation or expansion of the blood vessels to allow more blood to the skin for cooling. If we get too cold, our blood capillaries constrict and allow less blood to the surface of the skin. We sweat less, and the hair on our body stands up to trap more air. Our metabolism might even drop and cause us to start shivering. The system works to keep body temperature within a very narrow range.

It's the same with blood sugar. Levels of this critical nutrient are monitored by the pancreas and controlled by the hormone insulin, which instructs the cells to take up glucose out of the blood. This homeostatic system maintains blood glucose within a very narrow range.

Homeostasis also comes into play when we start to exercise. If you haven't exercised for some time, increased movement will shock your body, which will then shout at you to stop this abnormal activity. It will resist even harder the next time you try it. For example, suppose you put on your new workout outfit and head out the door. You start walking briskly down the street using your heart rate monitor to increase your heart rate gradually. At some point homeostasis kicks in. You might begin to feel nauseous, you might become short of breath, your muscles might feel uncomfortable, or you might suddenly feel weak. That's your body shouting, "What are you doing? This isn't normal. Normally you sit in front of the television this time of day. Stop right now and go home!" If you feel truly awful, you may obey that command. I call these messages "monkey talk." That's when imaginary monkeys sit on your shoulder, whispering things like, "It's okay to stop and go home. Exercise is not for you. You don't need to put yourself through this suffering. Go home and raid the refrigerator for a hot fudge sundae. Come on. Be nice to yourself." This is all part of homeostasis. It will happen when you first start to exercise, or when you attempt to step up your fitness levels, or when you try to alter your eating habits, lifestyle, or daily routine. But if you anticipate the "monkey talk," short-circuit it and accomplish the permanent changes you want to make in your life. All it takes is a strong dose of motivational magic.

Mobilizing Motivation

How do people like Jeanette overcome the body's wish to stay where it is now? As with all parts of the Fit *and* Fat program, it depends on an array of individual traits. We all possess different levels of motivation. Some of us are naturally more self-motivated than others. We explored this fact in Chapter 8, where you made accommodations in your personal fitness plan for your particular level of self-motivation. I wish I could prescribe a magic potion that would instantly give you superhuman motivation, but, of course, I can't. But I can teach you a few tricks I've picked up over a lifetime spent in the world of fitness.

When I turned 40, I set myself a fitness-training and racing goal: to set the Master's World Record at the Ironman Triathlon. When I accomplished that, I struggled to find a new fitness-training goal. Nothing lay beyond that world record, I thought. Lacking new tangible goals, I lost my motivation. My training became lackluster, my energy shifted, and I drifted. I searched inside my heart, asking, "What do I want to do? Why do I want to do it?" The answers came slowly but surely.

Ultimately, I decided to do the Ironman Triathlon again, but this time I would set the record in each of five major Ironman races around the world. It took a couple years, but I accomplished that goal. As I started to approach age 50, I had to search still deeper to find my goal. After all, what lies beyond the hardest races in the world? The answer came as I approached 50. I would match what I had achieved at 40: break the World Ironman record for women 50 years and over. I'll never forget the mental struggle it took for me to convince myself that I could do it.

I also found motivation and inspiration in a most unusual place. From the age of 40, I had spent 10 solid years finishing dead last in a yearly series of sprint-distance triathlons, the Danskin Triathlons for women, as the volunteer "final finisher." It was, and still is, a great job because I can ensure that no woman will ever suffer the agony of coming in last in the race. For many of the women I meet, just crawling to the finish line takes superhuman motivation. Meeting these women inspired me to get the fittest in my life, fit enough to accomplish even more challenging goals. When I started the Ironman training again; when I started to see my fitness levels improve week after week; when I started to see my body shape change as I got stronger, leaner, and faster, the improvement alone motivated me more. A magic wand waved over my metabolism, my physical powers, and my emotional states. Step by step, I slowly gained more and more ability—and the more I gained, the more motivated I felt. I love to train. I love to race. I was having the time of my life.

In fact, I was having such a grand time the year I turned 50 that I let it get the better of me. I had gotten so fit that I decided to compete in three big races that year: a 3,200-mile Bicycle Race Across America (RAAM) as part of a 4-woman relay team, a 4-day adventure race in China a month later, and the Ironman World Championships in Hawaii a month after that. I thought I could set the record in the Ironman because I was so fit. In reality, I was exhausted. Oh, I still completed the race faster than I had ever done it before, but I came in fourth.

After recovering from the race, I reviewed my performance and decided I had allowed myself to lose touch with my goal: I had let my ego and other goals distract me from the race that really mattered to me. So as you might expect, I decided to go back and do better: In my fifty-first year I would win the Grand Masters (50-and-over age class) at the Ironman Triathlon. I finished second in the race by just five minutes, losing to a wonderful woman named Lynn Brooks, but I had raced the fastest Ironman Triathlon of my life.

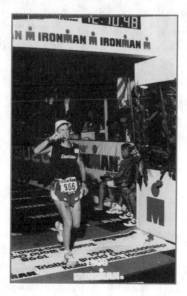

Sally Edwards finishing the Hawaii Ironman Triathlon at age 51.

People often ask me how I have motivated myself to keep training and racing at a high level for so many years. I chalk up some of my success to my genetics and some to the strong will pounded into me as the only girl in a family of boys with a strict military father. But I've also learned a lot over the years. The four most important lessons I can share with you are these:

- Master the art of setting yourself challenging yet realistic goals.
- Develop the skills to navigate obstacles, detours, and roadblocks.
- Maintain a high self-confidence and body image.
- Sustain yourself with the support of family and friends.

Although you may find my life as a professional athlete far removed from your own life and your struggles with fitness and fatness, we all can use these four skills to achieve what we want in life.

Setting the Right Goals

We've talked about the importance of goals, but now I'd like you to think about the ways in which goals help maintain your motivation. In the previous chapter, we discussed setting goals when you built your personal activity plan, exploring such topics as making your goals specific, creating a strategy for accomplishing them, keeping them sensible, and mastering the strength to keep going when the going gets tough. Here, however, I want to show you why fitness goals work better than weight-loss goals. The mere thought of weight loss often pumps fear into our hearts. To stay motivated, we must abandon fear, replacing it with desire. Fear will never motivate you the way desire can.

Abandoning Weight-Loss Goals

If you focus on weight loss as your supreme goal, you're setting yourself up for a fall. Why? Because chasing that goal distracts you from all the important changes you want to make in order to become physically, metabolically, and emotionally fit.

In our society the sayings "You can never be too rich" and "You can never be too thin" have never been so true. However, it's also never been so true that riches and thinness have never been so elusive and that the single-minded pursuit of either could make you a miserable, anorexic Scrooge. The American public spends $30 billion a year trying to achieve weight loss, and yet the rates of obesity keep rising, with 60 percent of adults in the United States now classified as overweight or obese. It's a real battle in a culture that acts against your chances of weight loss: Our society obsesses with food, food portions keep getting bigger, and we're too busy to engage in essential daily physical activity. So why not give up the pursuit of weight loss and set better and more achievable goals, ones that will guarantee better fitness?

The fear of fat now rivals the fear of death in our society. Fat is the new "F" word. In a recent study, researchers invited children between ages five and eight to look at photographs of children—one in a wheelchair, one hairless after cancer treatment, one from an unknown foreign nation, and one fat child. The researchers wanted to know who the viewers would least want for a friend. The most shunned photograph was the fat child.[1] I would bet that a majority of American women shown the same photos would react the same as these children.

Fear of fat. We hear "fat," and we can't think straight. We panic. And when we find ourselves in a sea of panic, we grab the nearest straw to stay afloat. That straw is dieting, but it won't keep you afloat—it will sink you. Only when you can set aside the panic, only when you abandon that highly promoted diet, can you begin to think more clearly. With clear thinking, you can examine your reasons for wanting to get thin. When you do, you might surprise yourself. Do you desire thinness, or do you really desire the ability to play with your children at the park and to walk up and down stairs—to run, to feel comfortable in an exercise class, or to enjoy an evening of line dancing? These are fitness goals, and achieving them might result in some weight loss, but what is certain is that you will become a healthier, happier person.

The Fear of Fat: Lorraine's Story

I was so hung up about my weight that I could not discuss it with anybody without my heart racing and afterward feeling so bad about myself that the bad feelings lasted for days. This happened at the doctor's office, with my friends and family, and at the gym. What was happening with my emotional response to the situation was quite simply disabling. It was so bad, it was like I had a stutter when I had to say my weight in pounds. I was truly embarrassed and ashamed. I knew it was really stupid and that really I should get over it, but years of being harassed about my weight, from the playground as a child to the doctor's surgery as an adult, had left me unable to deal with it.

One day I hit upon a really neat way of getting around the problem while I healed from it: I would express my weight in kilograms instead of pounds. It was a little trick that freed me from the fear of fat and helped me look at the issue more objectively: at last I could see the number for what it was, just a number on a scale rather than a measure of my worthiness. Don't underestimate the grip that the fear of fat can have on your life.

Another reason to eschew weight-loss goals is that your energy black box just might not be ready for you to drop body weight. The research has shown that even if you do diet religiously, sticking to a strict eating plan and calorie intake, you still might not lose all the weight you want to lose—and you will surely put on more weight once you stop the diet.

Finally, focusing on weight loss will make you miserable because weight-loss goals originate from deprivation, and deprivation delights no one. Fitness goals do not demand deprivation; they demand positive action. And action delights everyone. By setting goals that expand your capabilities, improve your health, and give you more energy, you'll be taking the road that always leads to success and could even take you places you never even dreamed you'd visit. They took Jeanette and Lorraine to marathons and triathlons. When you achieve your fitness goals, you automatically and beneficially alter your physiology. You might not recognize your new mental or physical self. You might not notice you weigh less. But you will discover the rewards of greater metabolic, emotional, and physical fitness.

Activity 9.1: Replacing Your Weight-Loss Goals with Fitness Goals

Overweight people naturally want to lose weight. We live in a society in which every fat person receives a constant barrage of messages that they must lose weight for their health, for their sex life, for their appearance, and for their success at work, as a parent, and as a human being. These are wonderful goals, but I hope you see that dieting will not guarantee them. Fitness will. If you've never really tried fitness, doing so now will cause a big shift in your physiology and not only help you lose weight, but help you keep it off in the long term. If you are a fitness participant already, then focusing on your fitness in a more methodical way will lead to changes that might or might not lead to weight loss. However, increasing your fitness will, I promise, give you the benefits of improved health and higher energy levels for parenting, your business, and your love life. Here's how you can replace your weight-loss goals with fitness goals:

1. Write down your weight-loss goal. For example, Lorraine initially wanted to lose 10 percent of her body weight and reduce her body fat percentage by 10 percent.

2. Force yourself to face your fear of fat. It's not easy, I know, but you can do it. Can you recall slurs or innuendoes from family, friends, or colleagues? Do

you remember childhood taunting, ridicule by the opposite sex when you were a teenager, or even physical or mental abuse from a family member?

Why do you want to lose weight? Are you concerned about your health? Do you worry about the way people see you? Does your fat prevent you from doing something you want to do? List these reasons in Column A of the table. A blank table is provided for you in Appendix F.

3. Now ask yourself, "Why is that a good reason to lose weight?" Will losing weight actually address the reason you state in Column A? For example, if you said you want to lose weight to enhance self-esteem, ask yourself if weight loss will really do that. Plenty of people of normal weight wrestle with self-esteem issues. And plenty of overweight people don't. Try to get to the bottom of why you want to lose weight. Write your answers in Column B.

4. Now you can consider how fitness can help you achieve what you thought you wanted to achieve through weight loss. Look at each of your reasons for weight loss in Column B. Write in Column C what else—especially fitness-oriented actions—you could do to help you address your need to lose weight.

5. Compare your notes in columns A and C. For example, Lorraine wanted to lose weight to improve her health. She learned that she could actually improve her health purely by focusing on her fitness (her resting heart rate, exercising heart rate, blood pressure, and levels of blood fats). She had thought her weight was holding her back from becoming a better mountaineer and from dressing well. In reality, fitness could help her become fitter for climbing mountains, and a bit of ingenuity could help her dress better. With a little mental effort, you should find the rationale you've built up over many years for weight loss to crumble before your eyes. Now you can replace it with a rationale for improved metabolic, emotional, and physical health. Well done.

Here's how Lorraine filled out the table:

A: Reasons why I want to lose weight:	B: Why is that a good reason to lose weight?	C: How else, using fitness or otherwise, could I address my vindication for my need to lose weight?
The doctors keep telling me to lose weight.	It's unhealthy to weigh as much as I do.	Actually, I could improve my health vastly by improving my fitness, without even losing any weight.

Activity 9.1. *continued*

A: Reasons why I want to lose weight:	B: Why is that a good reason to lose weight?	C: How else, using fitness or otherwise, could I address my vindication for my need to lose weight?
I want to get fit enough to be a better mountaineer.	If I could lose some weight, I could be fitter.	I could probably get fitter and become a better mountaineer by improving my fitness alone.
I'm fed up with not having the choice of clothes that slimmer women have.	If I had a wider choice of clothes, I would be happier. I could dress myself in a more attractive way.	There are actually lots of women who are larger and turn themselves out in a very attractive manner. I just need to be more imaginative and maybe search harder for styles and stores that suit me. Even thin women find it difficult to find clothes that suit them.
People find me imposing as a woman, and I'm sure it's something to do with my size.	If I were slimmer and more attractive, people wouldn't feel so intimidated.	Size is only part of being intimidating. Perhaps I need to focus on being more friendly, approachable, and easygoing.
I'm terrified of what will happen to my weight if I have a baby. Will I be huge? Will I be able to lose the weight afterward?	If I can't control my weight now, what hope have I got during pregnancy and afterward? Where will my fatness end?	That's not necessarily so. Fitness is something that will help me maintain a healthy weight during pregnancy, have an easier birth, and make a better recovery.

Overcoming Setbacks and Roadblocks

On your journey to improved health and fitness, you may occasionally run into obstacles, detours, or even setbacks. An illness, a pregnancy, a long trip away from home, an injury, or a crisis such as a divorce or a death in the family may occur, but when they do, they need not mean failure on the fitness front. We all must accept and cope with such events. They are not failures or inadequacies; they're just part of life's adventure. Over the years, I've discovered some techniques anyone can use to overcome setbacks and roadblocks.

The first technique is something I call "reframing." It's a process of changing the positive to the negative, redefining a half-empty cup as one that's half full. When you reframe, you turn your anxiety or fear of something into a desire, a pleasure, and a challenge. Reframing fortifies the positive and discards the negative.

If during your everyday activities an incident occurs that looks like a barrier, reframe it in nonstressful terms. For example, let's say the doctor called you today and left a message for you to return the call. If this event alarms you, then reframe it with a positive spin: He is just calling to remind you of an appointment. The energy generated by sheer optimism and positive thinking makes life brighter, even if bad news does arrive.

Using positive self-talk flips negative ideas into energizing ones. For example, if you say to yourself, "I dread doing my strength training today," reframe it as "I know it is important for me to do resistance workouts to build my muscle mass, and it is one of the things I really need to accomplish." Or, if you hear that inner voice, your "monkey mind," yakking away with the "I am too tired today" rap, reframe your inner conversation to "I know that once I get started, I'll feel happy to be working out." I use a trigger word whenever my mind engages in negative self-talk, saying "faido" to tell me to stop the negativity and replace it with positive affirmations. I took my trigger word from the Ironman race in Japan, where I finished second. There the spectators on the course yelled "Faido!" at us to keep us going. It means "to fight against that which is inside each of us that keeps us from doing our best."

Activity 9.2: Reframing

To practice reframing, let's play a little game. The most common excuses fitness participants give for not training are lack of time, lack of energy, and lack of motivation. Which of these could be your Achilles heel? Anticipating possible barriers is the first step toward conquering them. Look back, look at your life today, and look forward to identifying whatever has or might get in your way as you implement your program. List as many as you can.

Next, state the obstacle in negative terms and then reframe it in positive terms. For example, take a knee injury:

Fit *and* Fat

Activity 9.2. *continued*

Past, Present, or Future Roadblock	Negatively Stated	Positively Reframed
I injured my knee.	A knee injury stops me from running or cycling.	I will learn how to heal this injury and, more important, prevent it in the future. While my knee is healing I can do some emotional fitness training and some strength training.

Play the game for all the obstacles you have encountered or anticipate encountering. You will soon find yourself tapping the incredible power of positive thinking.

Here's how to reframe some of the most common roadblocks:

The Reframing Game

Past, Present, or Future Roadblock	Negatively Stated	Positively Reframed
I don't have enough time.	My lack of time is preventing me from working out and getting fitter.	It's only a matter of time management and setting priorities. I might be fat, but I'm not stupid, and I can manage my time better.
I don't know how to exercise properly.	I've never had the opportunities to learn what it is to participate in sports, so that's just the way I'll stay.	I've never had the opportunities, but it's not going to stop me going out now and making the opportunities. I can do this.
I don't have a program.	How can I do without a program? If somebody would give me a proper program, I might be able to attempt it.	I am the only person in control of my destiny. I have to make my own program. That's the best way.
I don't have a fitness-training partner.	Nobody wants to train with me—I'm too slow and too fat.	There are plenty of people my size who probably feel just the same way. If I hook up with

230

Past, Present, or Future Roadblock	Negatively Stated	Positively Reframed
		another person in the same situation, we'll both benefit. In fact, I could be doing somebody else a favor!
I don't have the right equipment.	I don't have the equipment, nor can I afford it. I'm not made of money.	Where there's a will, there's a way. I can start off with begged or borrowed equipment and then see what I really need later.
I don't have the right clothes.	Unless I spend a lot of money getting the right outfit, I'm going to stick out like a sore thumb, and that will make be feel worse about the whole thing. If I go ahead and purchase new stuff, I might be wasting my money if I quit.	Sometimes it's better to look like a beginner, which I am, than be labeled "All the gear, no idea." I can start with what I've got. People don't really care what you wear; it's only fashion, after all.
I get injured easily.	Whenever I start an exercise program, something happens to me. I'm just not built for it.	A common reason for injuries is going too hard too fast. If I regulate my intensity with my heart rate monitor, I should be able to stay injury-free. If one particular activity doesn't suit me, there are always alternatives.
I don't have a place to exercise.	It's not safe or practical for me to exercise where I live.	There are places that are safe and practical; since it's a free land, I'll go there to exercise instead.

Building Self-Confidence and Improving Body Image

Remember the children's book *The Little Engine That Could?* It tells the story of a bunch of clowns, giraffes, elephants, bears, and other animals that needed to go up and over the top of a mountain. Each time a train passed by, they asked for a ride over the top of the mountain, and each time they were turned down because the passing trains were too busy, or were already carrying a load of freight, or were just too fancy to haul such a troop of characters. Then one day, the Little Blue Engine came chugging by and stopped. The Little Engine agreed to give the troop a ride, but it was so small that it really struggled with all of the animals on board. The challenge seemed impossible. As the story goes, though, the Little Blue Engine huffed and puffed and repeated the mantra, "I think I can," until, to rousing cheers, it made it to the mountain top.

It tugged and pulled and pulled and tugged
And slowly, slowly, slowly they started off.
Puff, puff, chug, chug, went the Little Blue Engine.
"I think I can—I think I can—I think I can—I think I can—I think I can."[2]

Training (pun intended) can challenge you as much as the mountain challenged the Little Blue Engine. Some days, you just don't know if you can make it, as weariness, distractions, and rationalizations pile up: "I'm too tired, I have to go to a movie, I'll just do it another day."

To become a successful fitness engine, you need a lot of self-confidence and a supremely positive body image. Low levels of self-confidence can do more than anything else to hold us back, while unflagging belief can propel us up the steepest slopes.

High levels of self-confidence come from hard information. As the information accumulates, so does your confidence in your ability to succeed. This information comes from different sources: what people say, your own excitement and imagination, your energy black box's response to energy shifting, your growing physical strength, and all your past successes and failures.

Activity 9.3: Building Self-Confidence

Strong belief in yourself multiplies your chances of success. Have past fitness and weight-loss disasters undermined your self-confidence in the area of health and fitness? Make it different this time. With the Fit *and* Fat program, you'll be gaining the benefits of fitness, not of weight loss. Unlike weight-loss activities, the activities that you will take toward fitness bestow tangible and lasting benefits.

Believing that you can accomplish the tasks that put you on the path to fitness will help you start and stay on your program. To reinforce this belief, brainstorm what you have accomplished with your body in the past, achievements unrelated to weight loss. These might include having played a sport in school, having learned to drive, having made yourself a good lover, having raised a child, or having done anything physical, from walking around the block to running a 15k race. Recognize that your ability to accomplish each of these tasks proves your ability to tackle and succeed at the task of getting fit. Use the following format to help you construct some positive statements that will help you when your self-confidence wanes. Write your list of personal achievements in your fitness log.

I Think I Can, I Think I Can …

Physical Accomplishment	How I Can Use That to Build Self-Confidence Now
For example, Lorraine wrote: "I took part in a 2,000-mile charity bike ride and was one of the strongest cyclists."	That just goes to show that I do have great stamina and endurance. I can keep going longer than a lot of people I know. Imagine what I could do if I develop this.

Body Image

There might be some truth to the old saying "You are what you eat," but I think there's more truth in "You are what you see in your mind's eye." If you look in the mirror and see a fat, ugly person, you'll truly feel like one. If you see a fit and healthy person, you'll end up happy with yourself. Letting go of negative body images and living a life without concerns about your body in other people's eyes will free you to focus on getting fit and improving your health. What have you got to lose?

Let's play another game, one that transforms words that describe a negative body image into words that help motivate you to achieve your fitness goals.

Activity 9.4: Improving Your Body Image

Circle the word that you would use to describe your body, and then look at its positive counterpart. When you find yourself muttering a bad word about yourself, replace it with a good word. Maybe there are more words you can add to the list.

The Body Image Transformer

Bad Words I Say About Myself	Good Words I Will Say About Myself as I Get Fit
Fat	Fit
Lumpy	Smooth
Saggy	Tight
Slow	Quick
Lethargic	Energetic
Embarrassed	Proud
Unathletic	Sporty
Sad	Happy

Notice how the good words correspond to goals? If you keep these good words in mind, they'll motivate you to attain them.

Gathering Support

Research shows that people who gather a lot of social support for their fitness program will more likely achieve their fitness goals.[3] Most people prefer to train with others rather than alone, partly because our partners provide constant encouragement and help. It's more than mere companionship. Finding a training buddy, a partner, a friend, a colleague, a coach, a personal trainer, a club, an organization, a therapist, or anyone who supports your commitment to your health can make a huge difference in your ability to stick with the new plan. Try training with a group, preferably a small group. Enlist the support of others by letting them know your goal or sharing with them your desire to form new habits. Ask others for their support; don't just assume they know you need it.

Teamwork pays. Recent research has revealed some interesting facts about fitness support teams:[4]

- Ninety percent of fitness participants prefer group exercise environments.
- Training with a "team" of like-minded individuals provides enhanced camaraderie and accountability.
- Training in a group alleviates loneliness and boredom from training and thus reduces drop-out rates.
- The "gold standard" for fitness training is one-on-one workouts with a fitness professional because of the personal attention, learning process, and positive power of communication.

Activity 9.5: Go, Team!

Regardless of your sex, marital status, or living arrangement, you can find people out there who can support you in your quest for fitness. It's just a matter of identifying what you need and then finding the people to help you. Most will be delighted when you ask. In the first column of the next table, you'll see a list of the types of social support and help you may require. Not all of them may apply to you, and you may need something that doesn't appear on the list. Modify it, if necessary. The second column presents ideas about where to get that type of support. In the final column, you can fill in the names of people or organizations that might provide the support you need. Take some time to organize and assemble your team.

Team _____ (Your Last Name)

Support Type	Where to Get It	Who Shall I Ask?
Training team, club, or group	Look in your local community.	_____
Training partner or buddy	Ask all of your friends.	_____
Child care	Look to professional care, neighbors, friends, and family.	_____
Coach or trainer	Ask an organization for your sport or hobby, or search online.	_____

Activity 9.5. *continued*

Support Type	Where to Get It	Who Shall I Ask?
Somebody to support me at events	Ask your friends and family.	_____
A medical advisor	Approach your health insurance company or medical directory, or get a referral from friends and family.	_____
A psychologist or therapist	Approach your health insurance company or medical directory, or get a referral from friends and family.	_____
A mentor to help me track my progress	Find an older or more experienced person from your training team or health club.	_____
A sports-specific coach	Find out the governing body for the sport or activity, and look for a qualified coach.	_____
A life coach or counselor to help sort out emotional issues	Look online or ask your friends.	_____
A sports therapist	Look in the Yellow Pages or get a personal recommendation.	_____
A massage therapist	Ask your friends for a personal recommendation.	_____
An organization that provides information for people participating in my sport	Use the Internet.	_____

The Motivation Spiral

The motivation it takes to change from unfit to fit or from fit to fitter requires more than just time and effort. It takes an understanding of the motivation process. By definition, motivation is energy, positive energy that maintains drive toward a goal. I like to picture the motivation process with the Motivation Spiral. Imagine traveling in widening circles and along the way discovering different places that intrigue and inspire you. Take a few minutes to tour the Motivation Spiral.

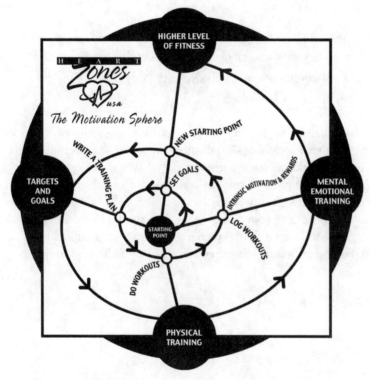

The Motivation Spiral.

Go from the starting point to the point when you set goals (small, attainable, action-oriented fitness goals that lead to improved health). Then move on to write a training plan. Do workouts and log workouts. Now you're reaping intrinsic motivation and rewards that propel you to a new starting point, a new plan, and a higher level of fitness. Although the diagram shows only one spiral, it really keeps expanding throughout your life. Each time you traverse a

Motivation Spiral, it gets bigger, you get fitter, and the training process becomes a more deeply ingrained habit.

Week 8 Summary

I opened this book with a message I hoped would motivate you to get fit, and I've closed it with the same message, providing real tools you can use to maintain your motivation. I talked about the natural resisting force of homeostasis. You can overcome this inertia with motivation. The secrets to maintaining motivation include these:

- Set yourself challenging yet realistic goals.
- Learn to navigate roadblocks, setbacks, detours, and obstacles.
- Build self-confidence and improve your body image.
- Gather support from others.

I also discussed the problems with weight-loss goals and gave you a tool for converting your weight-loss goals into fitness goals. To conquer setbacks and meet roadblocks on your journey to fitness, you can master the art of reframing, putting a positive spin on your reactions to obstacles. You need self-confidence and a positive body image to succeed. And you'll get more than mere support from your fitness team. You should be working out somewhere on the Motivation Spiral. Congratulations and good luck! We've reached the end of one trip together, but this is just the beginning.

Glossary

aerobic fitness   The ability of the body to maintain an exercise intensity while producing energy mainly from the aerobic metabolism.

anaerobic metabolism   Oxidation of carbohydrates without the ready availability of oxygen.

atherosclerosis   *See* arteriosclerosis.

athlete   A person who takes care of their health and fitness.

arteriosclerosis   A chronic disease involving loss of elasticity and thickening of the walls of the arteries.

biological makeup   The inherited genetic makeup that gives rise to biochemical individuality.

black box theory   A theory used to understand physical and biological systems where the mechanism is not yet understood.

blood fats   Lipids in the blood.

body mass index (BMI)   A mathematical formula that relates weight to height: (weight in kg ÷ [height in meters]^2).

bonk   A point of fatigue at which stored carbohydrates are depleted and an individual is limited in their ability to maintain a high steady exercise intensity. Also known as hitting the wall, knocking, or being overtaken by the person with the hammer.

carbohydrates   The energy-producing portion of food containing carbon, hydrogen, and water. Includes starches, glucose, and other sugars.

catecholamines   A group of hormones that work antagonistically with insulin to regulate fat burning.

ceiling   The top limit of a heart zone.

cholesterol   A hard, waxy substance produced mainly by the liver that is an essential component of cell membranes.

criss-cross workout   A workout that moves alternatively up and down through a range of heart beats.

Danskin   A New York City–based women's apparel company that sponsors a triathlon series.

delta heart rate   The difference between a heart rate measured in a prone or lying down position and a heart rate taken after a person has been standing still for two minutes.

diastolic blood pressure   The pressure in your arteries as your heart relaxes and fills with blood.

electrically measured heart rate   The speed at which the heart contracts, expressed in beats per minute (bpm), as measured using a heart rate monitor that picks up an electrical signal generated by a node in the heart that instructs the heart muscle to contract.

emotional fitness   The ability to deal with stress, build positive relationships, deal with change, and maintain a positive mental attitude.

energy black box   The energy-balancing mechanisms, which include the hormonal system, the nervous system, the brain, and the circulatory system, and regulate our energy levels, metabolism, and level of fatness and fitness, viewed from the perspective of the black box theory.

energy equation   The simple "energy in = energy out" equation used in the past to predict weight gain and loss.

energy shifting   A nondiet approach to balancing eating with metabolic, emotional, and physical fitness.

epinephrine   One of the catecholamine hormones that has an important role in promoting fat metabolism.

fat   A classification of overweight or obese according to BMI (body mass index) standards; someone with a high proportion of body fat according to an idealized standard; or anyone who thinks they are fat.

fat burning   Fat oxidation for energy production.

fat burning range   The range of heart beats over which fat is the principal source of energy.

fatty acids   The basic building blocks of fats.

floor   The bottom limit of a heart zone.

genetic heritage   A person's inherited genetic makeup.

glucose   A simple form of sugar.

glucose tolerance   The metabolism's ability to deal with inputs of glucose.

glucagon A hormone produced by the pancreas that aids in the breakdown of glycogen.

glycemic index (GI) A measurement of the immediate effect of different foods on blood glucose.

glycogen A storage form of glucose.

heart rate The number of beats or contraction cycles your heart makes per minute, measured by the electrical impulses emitted by your heart during this process.

heart zones A range of heart beats, usually 10 percent of your individual maximum, sport-specific heart rate. There are five different heart zones: Zone 1: 50 to 60 percent of maximum heart rate; Zone 2: 60 to 70 percent of maximum heart rate; Zone 3: 70 to 80 percent of maximum heart rate; Zone 4: 80 to 90 percent of maximum heart rate; Zone 5: 90 to 100 percent of maximum heart rate.

high-density lipoprotein (HDL) A chemical structure made up of a lipid and a protein to enable lipids (insoluble) to be transported in the blood. HDLs, as opposed to LDLs, have a low proportion of lipid compared to protein, which gives them a higher density—that is, they float less easily than LDLs.

homeostasis A natural feedback mechanism that maintains equilibrium. In the body, homeostatic mechanisms include heat regulation, blood glucose regulation, and hydration regulation.

insulin A hormone released by the pancreas that acts to lower blood glucose.

insulin sensitivity The responsiveness of the body's cells to insulin.

interval workout A type of workout where you alternate between very high heart rates or training intensities and low heart rates of rest periods.

intramuscular triglycerides Fats stored in and around the muscles.

Ironman A series of ultra-long-distance triathlon races.

lactate A chemical produced from the waste products of muscles undergoing intense exercise.

lipid An organic compound insoluble in water but soluble in organic solvents. Includes fatty acids, oils, and waxes.

low-density lipoprotein (LDL) A chemical structure made up of a lipid and a protein to enable lipids (insoluble) to be transported in the blood. LDLs, as opposed to HDLs, have a high proportion of lipid compared to protein, which gives them a lower density—that is, they float more easily than HDLs.

math max heart rate   The predicted heart rate as calculated using a mathe-matical equation.

max fat burning   The heart rate where fat is oxidized at the highest rate.

maximum heart rate   The greatest number of beats per minute possible for your heart. This number is highly individualized and is sport specific.

metabolic fitness   A health metabolism including healthy levels of blood fats, glucose tolerance, and blood pressure.

metabolism   The sum of all the chemical processes in the body resulting in energy production and growth.

norepinephrine   One of the catecholamine hormones that has an important role in promoting fat metabolism.

obese   A person's weight that is greater than 30 BMI (body mass index).

overweight   A person's weight that is greater than 25 BMI (body mass index).

pancreas   A gland near the stomach that supplies the duodenum with diges-tive fluid and secretes insulin into the blood.

PAR-Q (Participant Activity Readiness Questionnaire) test   A standard risk-assessment questionnaire that is used prior to involvement in physical activity. It was developed by the Canadian Society for Exercise Physiology.

peak heart rate   The highest heart rate reached during any single workout period.

physical fitness   A person's cardiovascular fitness, strength, and flexibility.

plasma triglycerides   Fats in the blood stream.

pulse   The rate at which you can feel the blood being pushed through your veins by the contractions of your heart. This is not the same as electrically measured heart rate.

recovery heart rate   The difference in the heart rate after an exercise session and after rest and commonly measured two minutes after stopping or slowing exercise.

resting heart rate   The number of heart beats per minute when the body is at complete rest.

steady state heart rate   A heart rate or training rate that is sub-maximal and maintained at a constant intensity, speed, or rate of work.

steady state workout   A type of workout in which you hold a steady heart rate for a sustained period of time.

stress response   The body's response to a perceived external threat, measured by heart rate, blood pressure, blood vessel constriction, and hormonal changes.

stressor   A demand on physical- or mental-energy, which is perceived as an external threat.

Syndrome X   A term coined by Gerald Reaven to describe a cluster of metabolic parameters that predict heart disease.

systolic blood pressure   The pressure in your arteries when your heart contracts.

triathlon   An athletic event involving three disciplines, usually swimming, cycling, and running.

triglyceride   The chemical name for a type of fat stored in the body.

type II diabetes   A chronic disease resulting from prolonged insulin resistance and overproduction of insulin by the pancreas. Onset of type II diabetes is defined by the failure of the pancreas to produce sufficient insulin.

visceral fat   Fat stored in the abdominal region in and around the vital organs.

VO_2   The volume of oxygen uptake or the capacity of the heart and lungs to supply oxygen to working tissues.

APPENDIX B

Maximum Heart Rate Test Protocol

Caution: The American College of Sports Medicine offers the following recommendation: Maximal effort testing performed by men over the age of 40 and women over the age of 50, even when no symptoms or risk factors are present, should be performed with physician supervision.

Heart Zones offers the following additional recommendation: A maximal stress test and health appraisal by a physician or sports physiologist is the safest way to determine your maximum heart rate.

Overview: The accurate assessment of your maximum heart rate results in the development of a precise, personalized fitness-training program because it sets the appropriate numbers for your specific five training heart zones. This test can be conducted by a trained exercise professional in a laboratory, in a club, or in the specific activity, or you can conduct the test yourself with another person assisting you.

During the assessment, you need to push yourself to your maximum effort for your current fitness level. This means that you need to go to the point of total effort. The test begins at an easy effort and progressively increases your pace and efforts until you reach a point that you are forced to slow down. It's only natural that this test creates some muscular pain, and it can be very uncomfortable. Terminate the test at any time if your breathing becomes impaired or you feel chest pains. Report this outcome to your medical professional.

Before you take the maximum heart rate test, complete all the submaximum tests to give you an indication of your maximum rate. These tests are all explained in this book (see Chapter 3). The test consists of 15-second stages with each stage increasing effort by 5 bpm until you are no longer able to increase your heart rate. The duration of the test should be between 2 and 4 minutes as you increase your effort by 5 bpm each 15 seconds. Before you begin and after you finish the test, warm up and cool down adequately. During the last 30 to 60 seconds of the test, your effort will be very strenuous, so men-tally prepare yourself for that in advance. Tighten the chest strap that attaches to the transmitter unit by one or two inches more than you normally have it to ensure a more accurate reading. Ask someone to assist you by providing you with the elapsed time, your heart rate data, and lots of encouragement. Train them in advance about the protocol and what they will be responsible for. You can do this test indoors or outdoors, doing any fitness activity, on most pieces of cardiovascular equipment—bicycle, treadmill, elliptical machine, etc.

Description: Before you begin the test, put on your heart rate monitor and tighten the chest strap. Start the heart rate reading function on the monitor. Set your watch so you can measure elapsed time.

Start the test with a complete warm-up, at least 5 minutes long and get-ting to but not exceeding a heart rate of 110 to 130 bpm or 60 percent of your estimated maximum heart rate from taking your sub-maximum assessments. Gradually increase the effort so your heart rate climbs approximately 5 beats every 15 seconds. At each 15-second interval, your assistant should ask you to look at your monitor and shout out the heart rate number so she can record it. Your assistant should also provide you with ongoing verbal encouragement throughout your workout. As your exercise intensity increases, your heart rate increases in a linear fashion as well until you reach a point that as you increase the effort to your maximum perceived exertion, your heart rate no longer increases. Record that heart rate number, the highest number that you experi-ence, and immediately begin your cooling down. A diagram of your test should resemble the following.

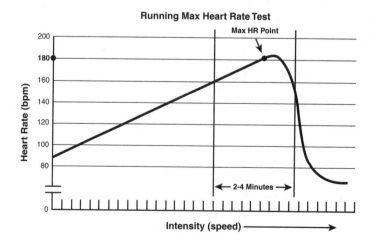

Running Max Heart Rate Test

246

Equipment needed:

- A heart rate monitor
- A watch that shows seconds
- A partner to assist you
- The form to record the data
- Facility or equipment on which to perform the test

Steps:

1. Warm up adequately for a minimum of 5 minutes in Zone 1.
2. After your warm-up, begin the test by increasing your effort by 5 bpm every 15 seconds.
3. Have your partner tell you your heart rate and the elapsed time every 15 seconds and record that information on the form.
4. Continue the test until your heart rate no longer increases although your effort does or until you can no longer continue because of fatigue.
5. Have your assistant verbally encourage your effort, especially at the end stages of the assessment.
6. Cool down slowly until you are comfortable and your heart rate is below 60 percent of your estimated maximum.
7. Use the highest number your monitor registered as your tested maximum heart rate.

Maximum Heart Rate Recording Form

Elapsed Time (minutes:seconds)	Heart Rate (bpm)
Warm up	_____
0 to 15	_____
15 to 30	_____
30 to 45	_____
45 to 60	_____
1:00 to 1:15	_____
1:15 to 1:30	_____
1:30 to 1:45	_____

Maximum Heart Rate Recording Form *(continued)*

Elapsed Time (minutes:seconds)	Heart Rate (bpm)
1:45 to 2:00	_____
2:00 to 2:15	_____
2:15 to 2:30	_____
2:45 to 3:00	_____
3:15 to 3:30	_____
3:30 to 3:45	_____
4:00 to 4:15	_____
4:15 to 4:30	_____
4:30 to 4:45	_____
4:45 to 5:00	_____

About Heart Zones

Dedicated to putting the heart back into emotional, metabolic, and physical fitness training, Heart Zones uses the heart and heart rate data to help individuals optimize their health. The company serves as the corporate network for dozens of different branded products, services, and programs such as Fit *and* Fat. Heart Zones hosts seminars, workshops, and certifications throughout the world as well as an annual international fitness conference. Details are easily available by logging onto www.heartzones.com.

Heart Zones Activities	Heart Zones Application Programs	Heart Zones Services	Heart Zones Global	Products
Seminars	Heart Zones Cycling	Coaching	Heart Zones Canada	Books
Workshops	Heart Zones Personal Training	Television	Heart Zones UK	Computer software
Certifications	Heart Zones Emotional Fitness Training	International		E-mail training
Conferences	Heart Zones Horse Training	Licensing		E-newsletter
Master Trainer Network	Heart Zones Fit *and* Fat			Program kits
Software development	Heart Zones Fitness Activities			Apparel
Branded products	Heart Zones School Education			Gear

Heart Zones Activities	Heart Zones Application Programs	Heart Zones Services	Heart Zones Global	Products
Licenses Heart Zones Health Clubs	Heart Zones Performance Camp			Educational charts
Content development				
Trade show participation				
Consulting				
Website activities				
New program development				

Resources

If you want to continue learning about fitness and fatness, here are some resources that will lead you to new equipment, friends, support networks, workout clothes, or sources of knowledge that will help you achieve your optimum level of health and fitness. Never stop learning, and never stop having fun.

To learn more about Heart Zones training, contact www.heartzones.com.

To purchase a heart rate monitor, log on to www.heartratemonitor.com.

To learn more about Fit *and* Fat, check out www.fitandfat.com.

Fitness Videos

The Fat Chick Works Out
Jeanette DePatie
www.thefatchick.com

In Fitness and in Health
Rochelle Rice
www.infitnessinhealth.com

In Grand Form
Jody Sandler
www.ingrandform.com

Move to Love Fitness
Linda Izzo
www.moretolovefitness.com

Fitness with Bliss
Kelly Bliss
www.kellybliss.com

Fitness Programs to Join

Feeling Good Fitness
415-869-2863
www.feelinggoodfitness.com

Low-impact, high-energy aerobics classes and personal fitness consulting/training by Jennifer Portnick, AFAA* Certified Aerobics Instructor and Personal Trainer in the San Francisco Area.

Bumblebee Fitness

www.bumblebeefitness.com

Personal trainer Sharon E. Snyder, ACE-certified Water Safety Instructor, specializing in plus-size fitness in the San Fransisco/Oakland/Berkeley areas.

New Face of Fitness

www.deehakala.com

A lifestyle program featuring exercise, support, behavior modification, and education. Founded by Dee Hakala. Several locations.

Big Moves

www.bigmoves.org

Dedicated to increasing size diversity in the world of dance. Offering dance classes. San Francisco area.

In Fitness and in Health

200 East 35th Street, Suite 2
New York, NY 10016
212-689-4558 or 1-877-943-7749
Fax: 212-447-6129
www.infitnessinhealth.com
info@infitnessinhealth.com

Exercise classes and health and fitness courses for large women leading an active life.

In Grand Form

604-984-9435 or 1-800-296-3077
Fax: 604-984-7828
www.ingrandform.com

Exercise classes, training courses for fitness professionals, using "at-your-size" approach in Vancouver area.

Sports Clothing

Danskin
www.danskin.com

A Big Attitude
www.abigattitude.com

Junonia
www.junonia.com

Alight.com
www.alight.com

Sports Equipment

Northwest Kayaks Inc.

www.nwkayaks.com

Offers a kayak called a Cadence that has a load capacity of 455 pounds and has an opening made for larger people.

Amplestuff

www.amplestuff.com

Serves the special needs of the millions of men and women who are plus-size or super-size. Offers products from extra wide socks to Ample-size bath towels.

The Greater Salt Lake City Clothing Company

www.gslcc.com

Ski wear for big, beautiful people and more!

Fat Acceptance Websites and Organizations

Big Fat Blog

www.bigfatblog.com

Internet discussion forum for fat acceptance, equality, and sizism.

The National Organization to Advance Fat Acceptance (NAAFA)

www.naafa.org

Body Image

Body Positive

www.bodypositive.com

Boosting body image at any size.

FAT?SO!

www.fatso.com

About Face

www.about-face.org/

Body Talk **Magazine**

www.bodytalkmagazine.com

Adios Barbie.com

www.adiosbarbie.com

Information and Training for Health-Care Professionals

First Do No Harm Program

www.msu.edu/~burkejoy

An alternative approach for helping clients with weight-related concerns at Michigan State University. Free online training material.

Hugs

www.hugs.com

Training to deliver nondiet programs and workshops by the lifestyle professional or educator. These programs and workshops are suitable for settings in private practice, hospitals, health centers, HMOs, workplaces, high schools, and more.

Healthy Weight Network

www.healthyweightnetwork.com

Information on dieting, the failure of weight-loss programs, eating disorders, obesity, overweight, size acceptance, diet quackery, and moving ahead with the nondiet health at any size paradigm.

Sporting Events

Clydesdale Triathlon Events

www.teamclydesdale.org

Enables athletes to compete in weight classes promoting fitness, camaraderie, and competition among larger athletes.

Danskin Women's Triathlon Series

www.danskin.com/triathlon/index.html

The largest and longest-running event in the history of multi-sport.

Further Resources

Plus Size Yellow Pages
www.plussizeyellowpages.com

Plus Size Plus
www.plus-size-plus.com

Large Directory
www.largedirectory.com

How to Contact Us

We invite you to join and become more involved in the Heart Zones Fit *and* Fat program by contacting us. Heart Zones leads seminars, workshops, and certifications on the Fit *and* Fat program throughout the world. We also host an annual international fitness training conference for those interested in a comprehensive experience. Led by co-authors Lorraine Brown and Sally Edwards, the Fit *and* Fat program provides people, fitness and health professionals, teachers, and others with tools and systems to effectively help individuals to live an active and healthy lifestyle.

Information is easily available on ways to become involved in the Fit *and* Fat program:

- Sign up for the Heart Zones e-newsletter, which gives the latest, up-to-date information, at our website: www.HeartZones.com.

- Participate in a seminar, workshop, or certification program offered by Heart Zones.

- Contact us about quantity pricing on *Fit* and *Fat* so you can provide copies for others.

- E-mail us your questions and inquiries at staff@HeartZones.com.

- Write to us about your experiences with the program at Heart Zones, 2636 Fulton Avenue, Suite #100, Sacramento, CA 95821, or call 916-481-7283.

- Attend our international fitness training conference to learn the complete program and earn an advanced certification.

- Communicate with others to let them know about and share your successes with the Fit *and* Fat program.

- Request the free trial version of ZONEware, the official software of the Heart Zones system.

- Find a health club and school near you that teaches its members and students the Heart Zones application, and participate in their program or recommend that they add it to their activities and curriculum.

- Ask us about our Fit *and* Fat coaching programs for you.

Heart Zones Fit and Fat Program
2636 Fulton Avenue, Suite #100
Sacramento, CA 95821 USA
916-481-7283
Fax: 916-481-2213
www.HeartZones.com
staff@HeartZone.com
Lorraine Brown, co-author, *Fit* and *Fat*
Sally Edwards, co-author, *Fit* and *Fat*

Forms

Chapter 2

Activity 2.4: Measure Your Heart Rate

Fit and Fat Heart Rate Log

Activity	Day 1	Day 2	Day 3	Day 4	Day 5	Day 6	Day 7	Better
Resting heart rate (bpm)	____	____	____	____	____	____	____	⇓
Delta heart rate (bpm)	____	____	____	____	____	____	____	⇓
Recovery heart rate (bpm)	____	____	____	____	____	____	____	⇑

⇑ *Higher is better.*
⇓ *Lower is better.*

Activity 2.6: Rockport One-Mile Fitness Walking Test

This test is just a rough estimate of your actual fitness, but it is a place to start. After about eight weeks of regular walking, test yourself again to check your progress. Over time, you'll find either that you can cover the mile faster or that your heart rate will be lower, or both.

To score your test, find the chart for your sex among the following, and then find your age range and your heart rate. If your exact pulse isn't shown, round it up or down to the nearest 10 beats.

Activity 2.6. *continued*

Here are the one mile walk times for low, medium, and high fitness levels.

Examples:

For example, if you are a 47-year-old man who walked the 1-mile course with a heart rate of 120 in 16 minutes, you would be at the moderate fitness level.

If you are a 33-year-old woman who walked the course with a heart rate of 150 in 17 minutes, 30 seconds, you would be at a moderate fitness level.

Women

Age	Heart Rate	Low Fitness	Moderate Fitness	High Fitness
20 to 29	110	>20:57	19:08–20:57	<19:08
	120	>20:27	18:38–20:27	<18:38
	130	>20:00	18:12–20:00	<18:12
	140	>19:30	17:42–19:30	<17:42
	150	>19:00	17:12–19:00	<17:12
	160	>18:30	16:42–18:30	<16:42
	170	>18:00	16:12–18:00	<16:12
30 to 39	110	>19:46	17:52–19:46	<17:52
	120	>19:18	17:24–19:18	<17:24
	130	>18:48	16:54–18:48	<16:54
	140	>18:18	16:24–18:18	<16:24
	150	>17:48	15:54–17:48	<15:54
	160	>17:18	15:24–17:18	<15:24
	170	>16:54	14:55–16:54	<14:55
40 to 49	110	>19:15	17:20–19:15	<17:20
	120	>18:45	16:50–18:45	<16:50
	130	>18:18	16:24–18:18	<16:24
	140	>17:48	15:54–17:48	<15:54
	150	>17:18	15:24–17:18	<15:24

Age	Heart Rate	Low Fitness	Moderate Fitness	High Fitness
	160	>16:48	14:54–16:48	<14:54
	170	>16:18	14:25–16:18	<14:25
50 to 59	110	>18:40	17:04–18:40	<17:04
	120	>18:12	16:36–18:12	<16:36
	130	>17:42	16:06–17:42	<16:06
	140	>17:18	15:36–17:18	<15:36
	150	>16:48	15:06–16:48	<15:06
	160	>16:18	14:36–16:18	<14:36
	170	>15:48	14:06–15:48	<14:06
60+	110	>18:00	16:36–18:00	<16:36
	120	>17:30	16:06–17:30	<16:06
	130	>17:01	15:37–17:01	<15:37
	140	>16:31	15:09–16:31	<15:09
	150	>16:02	14:39–16:02	<14:39
	160	>15:32	14:12–15:32	<14:12
	170	>15:04	13:42–15:04	<13:42

Men

Age	Heart Rate	Low Fitness	Moderate Fitness	High Fitness
20 to 29	110	>19:36	17:06–19:36	<17:06
	120	>19:10	16:36–19:10	<16:36
	130	>18:35	16:06–18:35	<16:06
	140	>18:06	15:36–18:06	<15:36
	150	>17:36	15:10–17:36	<15:10
	160	>17:09	14:42–17:09	<14:42
	170	>16:39	14:12–16:39	<14:12
30 to 39	110	>18:21	15:54–18:21	<15:54
	120	>17:52	15:24–17:52	<15:24

Fit *and* Fat

Activity 2.6. *continued*

Age	Heart Rate	Low Fitness	Moderate Fitness	High Fitness
	130	>17:22	14:54–17:22	<14:54
	140	>16:54	14:30–16:54	<14:30
	150	>16:26	14:00–16:26	<14:00
	160	>15:58	13:30–15:58	<13:30
	170	>15:28	13:01–15:28	<13:01
40 to 49	110	>18:05	15:38–18:05	<15:38
	120	>17:36	15:09–17:36	<15:09
	130	>17:07	14:41–17:07	<14:41
	140	>16:38	14:12–16:38	<14:12
	150	>16:09	13:42–16:09	<13:42
	160	>15:42	13:15–15:42	<13:15
	170	>15:12	12:45–15:12	<12:45
50 to 59	110	>17:49	15:22–17:49	<15:22
	120	>17:20	14:53–17:20	<14:53
	130	>16:51	14:24–16:51	<14:24
	140	>16:22	13:51–16:22	<13:51
	150	>15:53	13:26–15:53	<13:26
	160	>15:26	12:59–15:26	<12:59
	170	>14:56	12:30–14:56	<12:30
60+	110	>17:55	15:33–17:55	<15:33
	120	>17:24	15:04–17:24	<15:04
	130	>16:57	14:36–16:57	<14:36
	140	>16:28	14:07–16:28	<14:07
	150	>15:59	13:39–15:59	<13:39
	160	>15:30	13:10–15:30	<13:10
	170	>15:04	12:42–15:04	<12:42

Chapter 4

Activity 4.3: Taking Five Steps to Shift Your Energy

Step 2: Your Bag of Tricks

1. _____
2. _____
3. _____
4. _____
5. _____
6. _____
7. _____
8. _____
9. _____
10. _____

Step 3: Priority Game

(A) Tricks	(B) Effectiveness	(C) Difficulty	(D) Score	(E) Ranking
Energy Tricks	Potential Effectiveness (1 = not very; 5 = very	Implementation (1 = hard; 5 = easy)	Score (multiply columns 1 and 2)	Rank (highest number = highest priority)
_____	_____	_____	_____	_____
_____	_____	_____	_____	_____
_____	_____	_____	_____	_____
_____	_____	_____	_____	_____
_____	_____	_____	_____	_____
_____	_____	_____	_____	_____
_____	_____	_____	_____	_____
_____	_____	_____	_____	_____

Activity 4.3. *continued*

(A) Tricks	(B) Effectiveness	(C) Difficulty	(D) Score	(E) Ranking
Energy Tricks	Potential Effectiveness (1 = not very; 5 = very	Implemen- tation (1 = hard; 5 = easy)	Score (multiply columns 1 and 2)	Rank (highest number = highest priority)
_____	_____	_____	_____	_____
_____	_____	_____	_____	_____
_____	_____	_____	_____	_____
_____	_____	_____	_____	_____
_____	_____	_____	_____	_____

Final List of Prioritized Energy-Shifting Activities

Priority No.   Activity

1   _____

2   _____

3   _____

4   _____

5   _____

6   _____

7   _____

8   _____

9   _____

10 _____

Chapter 8

Activity 8.5: Setting Your Goals

The Five S's of Goal Setting

S1—Stakes

Ultimate goal: _____

Stake 1: _____

Stake 2: _____

Stake 3: _____

Stake 4: _____

Stake 5: _____

S2—Specificity

Stake 1: _____

Stake 2: _____

Stake 3: _____

Stake 4: _____

Stake 5: _____

S3—Strategy

Stake 1: _____

Stake 2: _____

Stake 3: _____

Stake 4: _____

Stake 5: _____

S4—Sensibility

Stake 1: _____

Stake 2: _____

Stake 3: _____

Stake 4: _____

Stake 5: _____

S5—Strength

_____

Activity 8.6: Completing Your Personal Fitness Plan Profile

Personal Fitness Plan Profile

Activity	Your Results	Elements to Include in Your Fitness Program		
The five steps of fitness change (Activity 8.1)	_____	_____	_____	_____
Self-motivation inventory (Activity 8.2)	_____	_____	_____	_____
Forecasting the the odds (Activity 8.3)	Friends ___ Self-belief ___	_____ _____ _____	_____ _____ _____	_____ _____ _____
	Support ___	_____ _____	_____ _____	_____ _____
	Smoking ___	_____ _____	_____ _____	_____ _____
	Discomfort ___	_____ _____	_____ _____	_____ _____

Activity	Your Results	Elements to Include in Your Fitness		
Program	Body image ___	_____ _____ _____	_____ _____ _____	_____ _____ _____
Identifying priorities (Activity 8.4)	Metabolic training: _____ percent of my time Emotional training: _____ percent of my time Physical training: _____ percent of my time			

Activity 8.7: Building Your Own Fit *and* Fat Personal Activity Program

1. **Set the time.** How much time can you devote to working toward your goal per week?

    i) The number of days a week I can train: _____

    ii) The amount of time I can devote to training each day: _____

    My total weekly training time i) × ii) = _____

2. **Manage your time.** Look at your results from Activity 8.4. Divide your total amount of time among metabolic, emotional, and fitness training according to your priorities.

Type of Fitness Training	Percent of Your Time to Allocate to This Type of Training	Actual Time Allocated to This Type of Training
Metabolic fitness	___ percent	___ hours
Emotional fitness	___ percent	___ hours
Physical fitness	___ percent	___ hours

3. **Select your activities.**

Type of Fitness Training	Activities
Metabolic fitness	_____
	_____
	_____
Physical fitness	_____
	_____
	_____
Emotional fitness	_____
	_____
	_____

Activity 8.7. *continued*

4. **Choose the best time.**

Type of Fitness Training	Selected Activities	Schedule
Metabolic	_____	_____
	_____	_____
	_____	_____
Physical	_____	_____
	_____	_____
	_____	_____
Emotional	_____	_____
	_____	_____
	_____	_____

5. **Assemble your program.**

Weekly Fit *and* Fat Personal Activity Program

Day	Time	Workout	Additional Details: Type of Workout, Where, with Whom, Any Special Notes	Log: How Was the Workout?
Monday	_____	_____	_____	_____
	_____	_____	_____	_____
Tuesday	_____	_____	_____	_____
	_____	_____	_____	_____
Wednesday	_____	_____	_____	_____
	_____	_____	_____	_____
Thursday	_____	_____	_____	_____
	_____	_____	_____	_____
Friday	_____	_____	_____	_____
	_____	_____	_____	_____
Saturday	_____	_____	_____	_____
	_____	_____	_____	_____
Sunday	_____	_____	_____	_____
	_____	_____	_____	_____

Chapter 9

Activity 9.1: Replacing Your Weight-Loss Goals with Fitness Goals

A: Reasons why I want to lose weight:	B: Why is that a good reason to lose weight?	C: How else, using fitness or otherwise, could I address my vindication for my need to lose weight?
_____	_____	_____
_____	_____	_____
_____	_____	_____
_____	_____	_____
_____	_____	_____
_____	_____	_____
_____	_____	_____
_____	_____	_____

Activity 9.2: Reframing

Past, Present, or Future Roadblock	Negatively Stated	Positively Reframed
_____	_____	_____
_____	_____	_____
_____	_____	_____
_____	_____	_____
_____	_____	_____
_____	_____	_____
_____	_____	_____
_____	_____	_____
_____	_____	_____

Notes

Chapter 1

1. Gaesser, Glenn A. *Big Fat Lies*. New York: Fawcett Columbine, 1996.

2. Bouchard, Claude, ed. *Introduction to Physical Activity and Obesity*. Human Kinetics Publishers, Inc., 2000.

3. See note 2 above.

4. See note 2 above.

5. CNN.com. July 18, 2001. Posted 8:51 A.M. EDT (12:51 GMT) "U.S. Scientist: Fat Can Be Healthy."

6. See note 5 above.

7. Colles, Lisa. *Fat: Exploding the Myths*. Carlton Books Limited, 1998.

8. Wei, Ming, James B. Kampert, Carolyn E. Barlow, Milton Z. Nichaman, Larry W. Gibbons, Ralph S. Paffenbarger, and Steven N. Blair. "Relationship Between Low Cardiorespiratory Fitness and Mortality in Normal-Weight, Overweight, and Obese Men." *JAMA* 282 (1999): 1547–1553.

9. Lee, Chong Do, Steven Blair, and Andrew Jackson. "Cardiovascular Fitness, Body Composition, and All-Cause and Cardiovascular Disease Mortality in Men." *American Journal of Clinical Nutrition* 69 (1999): 373–380.

10. Paffenbarger, R. S. Jr., R. T. Hyde, A. L. Wing, and C. C. Hsieh. "Physical Activity, All-Cause Mortality, and Longevity of College Alumni." *New England Journal of Medicine* 314 (1986): 605–613.

11. Blair, Steven N., and Suzanne Brodney. "Effects of Physical Inactivity and Obesity on Morbidity and Mortality: Current Evidence and Research Issues." *Medicine and Science in Sports and Exercise* 31 (11) (1999): S646–S662.

12. Blair, Steven N., and Claude Bouchard, co-chairs. "Physical Activity and Obesity: American College of Sports Medicine Consensus Conference." *Medicine and Science in Sports and Exercise* 31 (1999): S497.

[13] National Institutes of Health and National Heart, Lung, and Blood Institute. "Clinical Guidelines on the Identification, Evaluation, and Treatment of Overweight and Obesity in Adults: The Evidence Report." *Obesity Research* 6 (Supplement 2) (1998): 51S–209S.

[14] See note 11 above.

[15] Myers, J., M. Prakash, V. Froelicher, D. Do, S. Partington, and J. E. Atwood. "Exercise Capacity and Mortality Among Men Referred for Exercise Testing." *New England Journal of Medicine* 346 (2002): 793–801.

Chapter 2

[1] Bryant, C. X., J. A. Peterson, and T. P. Sattler. "The Weight Game." *Fitness Management* (April 1999): 38.

[2] Booth, F. W., M. V. Chakravarthy, and E. E. Spangenburg. "Exercise and Gene Expressions: Physiological Regulation of the Human Genome Through Physical Activity." *Journal of Physiology* 543 (2) (2002): 399–411.

[3] Booth, F. W., M. V. Chakravarthy, S. E. Gordon, and E. E. Spangenburg. "Waging War on Physical Inactivity: Using Modern Molecular Ammunition Against an Ancient Enemy." *Journal of Applied Physiology* 93 (1) (2002): 3–30.

[4] National Institutes of Health and National Heart, Lung, and Blood Institute. "Clinical Guidelines on the Identification, Evaluation, and Treatment of Overweight and Obesity in Adults: The Evidence Report." *Obesity Research* 6 (Supplement 2) (1998): 51S–209S.

[5] Gaesser, Glenn A. *Big Fat Lies: The Truth About Your Weight and Your Health*. New York: Fawcett Columbine, 1996.

Chapter 3

[1] Brown, Jim, ed. "Maximum Heart Rate: Is 'The Formula' Useless?" *Georgia Tech Sports Medicine and Performance Newsletter* 9 (9) (June 2002): 1–2.

[2] Robergs, Robert A., and Roberto Landwehr. "The Surprising History of the 'HRmax = 220 – Age' Equation." *Journal of Exercise Physiology* 5 (2) (2002): 1–10.

Chapter 4

[1] Frank, Arthur. "Futility and Avoidance: Medical Professionals in the Treatment of Obesity." *Journal of the American Medical Association* 269 (16) (1993): 2132–2133.

[2] Young, Lisa R., and Marion Nestle. "The Contribution of Expanding Portion Sizes to the U.S. Obesity Epidemic." *American Journal of Public Health* 92 (2002): 246–249.

[3] Snyder, Ann C. *Exercise, Nutrition, and Health.* Traverse City, Michigan: Cooper Publishing Group, LLC, 1998.

[4] Alpert, S. "Growth, Thermogenesis, and Hyperphagia." *American Journal of Clinical Nutrition* 52 (1990): 784–792.

[5] Salbe, Arline D., and Eric Ravussin. "The Determinants of Obesity," in *Physical Activity and Obesity.* Claude Bouchard (ed). Champaign, IL: Human Kinetics, 2000.

[6] Colles, Lisa. *Fat: Exploding the Myths.* Carlton Books Limited, 1998.

[7] Jonas, Steven, and Linda Konner. *Just as You Are: How to Be Healthy Whatever Your Weight.* New York: Barnes and Noble Books, 2000.

[8] Jonas, Steven. 2002. E-mail to author, October 25, 2002.

[9] Foster, Carl. 2002. E-mail to author October 16, 2002.

Chapter 5

[1] Budd, Martin L. *Why Can't I Lose Weight?* London: Thorsons, 2002.

[2] Reaven, Gerald M., Terry Kristen, and Barry Fox. *Syndrome X: Overcoming the Silent Killer That Can Give You a Heart Attack.* New York: Fireside, 2000.

[3] Yam, D. "Insulin-Cancer Relationships: Possible Dietary Implication." *Medical Hypotheses* 38 (1992): 111–117.

[4] See note 2 above.

[5] Gaesser, Glenn A. *Big Fat Lies: The Truth About Your Weight and Your Health.* New York: Fawcett Columbine, 1996.

[6] See note 2 above.

[7] Fenn, Christine. *The Energy Advantage.* San Francisco: Thorsons, 1997.

[8] Libby, Peter. "Atherosclerosis: The New View." *Scientific American* (May 2002): 28–35.

[9] Devlin, J. T., M. Hirshman, E. D. Horton, et al. 1987. "Enhanced Peripheral and Splanchnic Insulin Sensitivity in NIDDM Men After Single Bout of Exercise." *Diabetes* 36 (1987): 434–439.

[10] Heath, G. W., J. R. Gavin, J. M. Hinderliter, et al. "Effects of Exercise and Lack of Exercise on Glucose Tolerance and Insulin Sensitivity." *Journal of Applied Physiology* 55 (1983): 628–634.

[11] Charatan, Fred. "Exercise and Diet Reduce Risk of Diabetes, U.S. Study Shows. *British Medical Journal* 323 (2002): 359.

[12] National Institutes of Health. "Consensus Development Conference on Diet and Exercise in Non–Insulin-Dependent Diabetes Mellitus." *Diabetes Care* 10 (1987): 639–644.

[13] Burnstein, R., C. Polychronakos, C. J. Toews, J. D. MacDouglas, H. J. Guyda, and B. I. Pasner. "Acute Reversal of the Enhanced Insulin Action in Trained Athletes: Association with Insulin Receptor Changes." *Diabetes* 34 (1985): 756–760.

[14] Crouse, S. F., B. C. O'Brien, J. J. Rohack, R. C. Lowe, J. S. Green, H. Toldon, and J. L. Reed. "Changes in Serum Lipids and Apolipoproteins After Exercise in Men with High Cholesterol: Influence of Intensity." *Journal of Applied Physiology* 79 (1995): 279–286.

[15] Shepherd, R. J. "What Is the Optimal Type of Physical Activity to Enhance Health?" in *Benefits and Hazards of Exercise*. Domhnall MacAuley, ed. London: BMJ Books, 1999.

[16] Stefanick, M. L. "Physical Activity for Preventing and Treating Obesity-Related Dilipidoproteinemias." *Medicine and Science in Sports and Exercise* 31 (1999): S609–S618.

[17] Déprés, Jean-Pierre, and Benoît Lamarche. "Low-Intensity Endurance Exercise Training, Plasma Lipoproteins, and the Risk of Coronary Heart Disease." *Journal of Internal Medicine* 236 (1994): 7–22.

[18] Kraus, W. R., J. A. Houmard, B. D. Duscha, K. J. Knetzger, M. B. Wharton, J. S. McCartney, C. W. Bales, S. Hene, G. P. Samsa, J. D. Otvos, K. R. Kulkarni, and C. A. Slentz. "Effects of the Amount and Intensity of Exercise on Plasma Lipoproteins." *New England Journal of Medicine* 347 (2002): 1483–1492.

19 Fagard, Robert H. "Exercise Characteristics and the Blood Pressure Response to Dynamic Physical Training." *Medicine and Science in Sports and Exercise* 33 (6) (2001): S484–S492.

20 Carrol, J. F., and C. K. Kyser. "Exercise Training in Obesity Lowers Blood Pressure Independent of Weight Change." *Medicine and Science in Sports and Exercise* 34 (4) (2002): 596–601.

21 Wolever, T. M., and C. Mehling. "High-Carbohydrates Low-Glycemic Dietary Advice Improves Glucose Disposition Index in Subjects with Impaired Glucose Tolerance." *British Journal of Nutrition* 87 (5) (2002): 477–487.

22 Hooper, Lee, Carolyn D. Summerbell, Julian P. T. Higgins, Rachel L. Thompson, Nigel E. Capps, George Davey Smith, Rudolph A. Riemersma, and Shah Ebrahim. "Dietary Fat Intake and Prevention of Cardiovascular Disease: A Systematic Review." *British Medical Journal* 322 (2001): 757–763.

23 Institute of Medicine of the National Academies. *Dietary References Intakes for Energy, Carbohydrates, Fiber, Fat, Protein, and Amino Acids (Macronutrients)*. Washington, D.C.: The National Academies Press, 2002.

Chapter 6

1 Collinge, William B., and Len Duhl. *The American Holistic Health Association's Complete Guide to Alternative Medicine*. Warner Books, 1997.

2 Gaesser, Glenn A., and Karla Dougherty. *The Spark: The Revolutionary New Plan to Get Fit and Lose Weight: 10 Minutes at a Time*. New York: Fireside, 2002.

3 Swain, D. P., and B. A. Franklin. "VO$_2$ Reserve and the Minimal Intensity for Improving Cardiorespiratory Fitness." *Medicine and Science in Sports and Exercise* 34 (1) (2002): 152–157.

4 Byrne, Nuala M., and Andrew P. Hills. "Relationships Between HR and VO$_2$ in the Obese." *Medicine and Science in Sports and Exercise* 34 (9) (2002): 1419–1427.

5 Powers, Scott, and Stephen Dodd. *Total Fitness: Exercise, Nutrition, and Wellness*. Boston: Allyn and Bacon, 1999.

Chapter 7

[1] Romijn, A. A., S. Klein, E. F. Coyle, L. S. Sidossis, and R. R. Wolfe. "Strenuous Endurance Training Increases Lipolysis and Triglycerides-Fatty Acid Cycling at Rest." *Journal of Applied Physiology* 75 (1) (1993): 108–113.

[2] See note 1 above.

[3] Spriet, L. L. "Regulation of Skeletal Muscle Fat Oxidation During Exercise in Humans." *Medicine and Science in Sports and Exercise* 34 (9) (2002): 1477–1484.

[4] Jeukendrup, A. E., W. H. M. Saris, and A. J. M. Wagenmakers. "Fat Metabolism During Exercise: A Review—Part II: Regulation of Metabolism and the Effects of Training." *International Journal of Sports Medicine* 19 (1998): 293–302.

[5] Martin, W. H. III, and S. Klein. "Use of Endogenous Carbohydrate and Fat as Fuels During Exercise." *Proceedings of the Nutrition Society* 57 (1998): 49–54.

[6] Jansson, E., and L. Kaijser. "Substrate Metabolism and Enzymes in Skeletal Muscle of Extremely Endurance-Trained Men." *Journal of Applied Physiology* 62 (3) (1987): 999–1005.

[7] Friedlander, A. L., A. C. Gretchen, M. A. Horning, T. F. Buddinger, and G. A. Brooks. "Effects of Exercise Intensity and Training on Lipid Metabolism in Young Women." *American Journal of Physiology* 275 (1998) (*Endocrinology Metabolism* 38): E853–E863.

[8] Phillips, S. M., H. J. Green, M. A. Tarnopolsky, G. J. F. Heigenhauser, R. E. Hill, and S. M. Grant. "Effects of Training Duration on Substrate Turnover and Oxidation During Exercise." *Journal of Applied Physiology* 81 (5) (1996): 2182–2191.

[9] Van Aggel-Leijssen, Dorien P. C., Wim H. M. Saris, Anton J. M. Wagenmakers, Joan M. Sendon, and Marleen A. Van Baark. "Effect of Exercise Training at Different Intensities on Fat Metabolism in Obese Men." *Journal of Applied Physiology* 92 (3) (2002): 1300–1309.

[10] Schrauwen, Patrick, Dorien P. C. van Aggel-Leijssen, Gabby Hul, Anton J. M. Wagenmakers, Hubert Vidal, Wim H. M. Saris, and Marleen A. van Baark. "The Effect of a 3-Month Low-Intensity Endurance Training Program on Fat Oxidation and Acetyle-CoA Carboxylase-2 Expression." *Diabetes* 51 (2002): 2220–2226.

11 Achten, J., M. Gleedson, and A. E. Jeukendrup. "Determination of the Exercise Intensity That Elicits Maximal Fat Oxidation." *Medicine and Science in Sports and Exercise* 34 (1) (2002): 92–97.

12 See note 11 above.

13 Byrne, N. M., and A. P. Hills. "Relationships Between HR and VO_2 in the Obese." *Medicine and Science in Sports and Exercise* 34 (9) (2002): 1419–1427.

Chapter 8

1 Bouchard, Claude. "Individual Differences in the Response to Regular Exercise." *International Journal of Obesity* 19 (S:4) (1995): S5–S8.

2 Bouchard, Claude, and Tuomo Rankinen. "Individual Differences in Response to Regular Physical Activity." *Medicine and Science in Sports and Exercise* 33 (6) (2002): S446–S451.

3 Locke, E. A., and G. O. Latham. "The Application of Goal Setting to Sports." *Journal of Sport Psychology* 7 (1985): 205–222.

Chapter 9

1 Walker, Philip. *"Fit versus Fat: What's Weight Got to Do with It?"* (online) IDEA Health and Fitness, Inc. Available at ideafit.com/fit_vs_fat.htm, 2001.

2 Piper, Watty. *The Little Engine That Could.* New York: Platt and Munk, 1930.

3 Wing, R. R., and J. M. Jakicic. "Changing Lifestyle: Moving from Sedentary to Active," in *Physical Activity and Obesity.* Claude Bouchard, ed. New York: Human Kinetics, 2000.

4 Annesi, James J. *Enhancing Exercise Motivation: A Guide to Increasing Fitness Center Member Retention.* Los Angeles: Leisure Publications, 1996.

Index

Index

Index

Index

285

Index

About the Authors

Sally Edwards has been a professional speaker for the past 20 years, with more than 500 speeches, seminars, workshops, and presentations. This is her tenth year as the national spokesperson for Danskin. Sally has finished 16 Ironman Triathlons and is a Masters world record holder. She has also competed in two Eco-Challenge Adventure races and in Olympic Marathon Trials; was Silver Medalist in the 1998 Master's World Games; was a winning team member in the Race Across America (3,100-mile bicycle race); and is a winner of the Iditashoe 100-Mile Snowshoe Race, the Western States 100-Mile Run, and the American River 50-Miler. She is the author of 18 books on sports and fitness, including *Heart-Zone Training* and the *Heart Rate Monitor Guidebook*.

A native of the United Kingdom, **Lorraine Brown** holds a Masters of Science degree. As a trained scientist, she has delved into the latest research on fitness and fatness. Once fat and unfit herself, she discovered the benefits of using a heart rate monitor and Heart Zones Training to get fit, become an athlete, and compete in triathlons and marathons. Qualified as a Group Fitness Instructor with the American Council on Exercise and an avid participant in sports and outdoor activities, Lorraine brings both hard science and personal experience to the subjects of overcoming the fear of fat, understanding true fitness, learning the language of the heart, conquering motivational hurdles, escaping from the mind-set of a "fat person," and living a healthy, happy life.

Cover photos: Emre Kucur
Charlie Wielski / brightroom